Volume 1

Pocket Atlas of Cross-Sectional Anatomy

Computed Tomography and Magnetic Resonance Imaging

Volume 1:
Head, Neck, Spine and Joints

Torsten B. Möller and Emil Reif

Translated by Clifford Bergman

388 Illustrations

1994
Georg Thieme Verlag Stuttgart · New York
Thieme Medical Publishers, Inc. New York

Dr. Torsten B. Möller
Dr. Emil Reif
Am Caritas-Krankenhaus
66763 Dillingen/Saar
Germany

Clifford Bergman, M.D.
Eglingerstr. 10
82544 Moosham
Germany

This book is an authorized and adapted translation of the German edition published and copyrighted 1993 by Georg Thieme Verlag, Stuttgart, Germany. Title of the German edition: Taschenatlas der Schnittbildanatomie.

Some of the product names, patents and registered designs referred to in this book are in fact registered trademarks or proprietary names even though specific reference to this fact is not always made in the text. Therefore, the appearance of a name without designation as proprietary is not to be constructed as a representation by the publisher that is in the public domain.

© 1994 Georg Thieme Verlag,
Rüdigerstraße 14, 70469 Stuttgart
Germany
Thieme Medical Publishers, Inc., 381 Park Avenue South, New York, N.Y. 10016

Typesetting by Fotosatz Froitzheim,
53113 Bonn
Printed in Germany by Karl Grammlich,
72124 Pliezhausen

ISBN 3-13-125501-3 (GTV, Stuttgart)
ISBN 0-86577-510-9 (TMP, New York)

Library of Congress
Cataloging-in-Publication-Data

Möller, Torsten B.:
Pocket atlas of cross sectional anatomy : computed tomography and magnetic resonance imaging / Torsten B. Möller and Emil Reif. Transl. by Clifford Bergman. – Stuttgart : New York : Thieme : New York : Thieme Med. Publ.

Dt. Ausg. u.d.T.: Möller, Torsten B.:
Taschenatlas der Schnittbildanatomie
NE: Reif, Emil;
Vol. 1. Head, neck, spine, and joints. – 1994

Dedicated to the American part of our roots
the
Riegner Family, Michigan
and
Ronge Family, Connecticut

Preface

This atlas presents the basic anatomy needed to interpret CT and MR images.

Diagnosis with cross-sectional images requires an adaption in thinking, even among experienced clinicians, to this specific form of anatomy. For this reason, this atlas presents both of the currently most important cross-sectional imaging technologies.

One of the reasons these techniques play such a significant role today is that they afford a very high resolution. Therefore it was important to us that this book remain compact and concise, in spite of its comprehensiveness in including all anatomic structures. The four-color illustrations were essential to this success.

The two volumes are each halves of a whole work, which is organized along strict lines: each image is accompanied by a color-coded diagram, which we drew ourselves to avoid inaccuracies. Schematic drawings showing the level of the cross section completes the spectrum of information necessary to interpret the image.

All images were done on patients or volunteers. For their ongoing support during the creation of this book, we thank our radiologic technicians and assistants, especially Michalea Knittel, Pia Saar, Gisela Wagner, Monjuri Paul, and Andrea Britz. The manuscript was typed by Helga Brettschneider and Gabi Müller. Special thanks to Dr. Markus Bach, Dr. Patrick Rosar, and especially Dr. Beate Hilpert for reading the manuscript and making helpful suggestions.

Dillingen, September 1993   Torsten B. Möller and Emil Reif

Table of Contents

Cranial CT, axial (canthomeatal) 2
Cranial CT, vessels (axial) 26
Petrous pyramid CT, axial 30
Cranial MRI, axial (horizontal plane) 36
Cranial MRI, vessels (axial) 68
Cranial MRI, sagittal 72
Cranial MRI, vessels (axial) 84
Cranial MRI, coronal (frontal) 86
Cranial MRI, vessels (coronal) 110
Neck, axial 114
Larynx, axial 139
Neck, sagittal 138
Neck, coronal 152
Spine, axial 170
Spine, sagittal 172
Temporomandiubular joint, sagittal 178
Shoulder joint, axial 180
Shoulder joint, sagittal 186
Shoulder joint, coronal 192
Hip joint, coronal 198
Knee joint, sagittal 204
Knee joint, coronal 216
Foot, sagittal 222
Foot, coronal 228
References 234
Index 235

Cranial CT

Cranial MRI

Neck

Spine

Musculoskeletal system

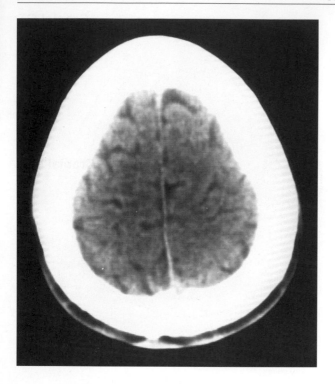

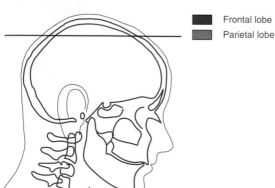

■ Frontal lobe
■ Parietal lobe

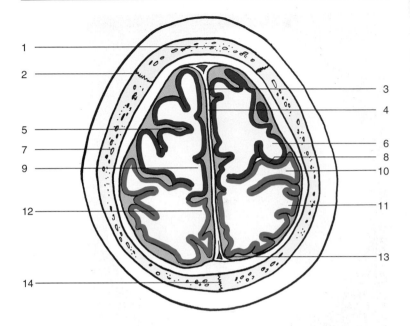

1 Frontal bone
2 Coronal suture
3 Longitudinal fissure
4 Falx of cerebrum
5 Precentral sulcus
6 Precentral gyrus
7 Parietal bone

8 Central sulcus
9 Paracentral lobule
10 Postcentral gyrus
11 Superior parietal lobule
12 Precuneus
13 Superior sagittal sinus
14 Sagittal suture

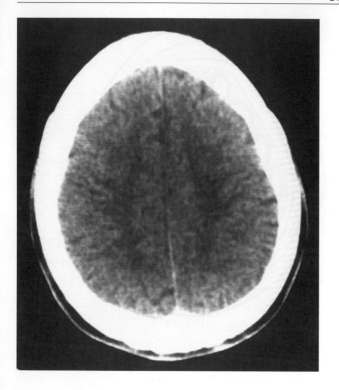

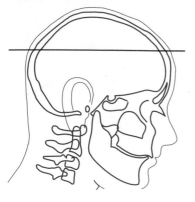

■ Frontal lobe
■ Parietal lobe

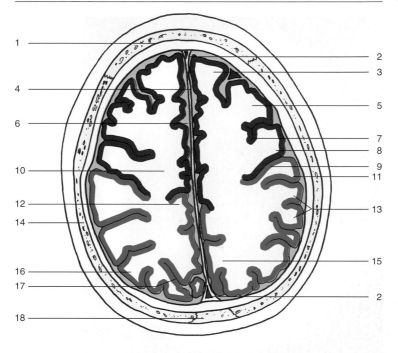

1 Frontal bone
2 Superior sagittal sinus
3 Superior frontal gyrus
4 Falx of cerebrum
5 Middle frontal gyrus
6 Longitudinal fissure
7 Precentral sulcus
8 Precentral gyrus
9 Central sulcus

10 Semioval center
11 Postcentral gyrus
12 Paracentral lobule
13 Supramarginal gyrus
14 Parietal bone
15 Precuneus
16 Inferior parietal lobule
17 Parietooccipital sulcus
18 Occipital bone

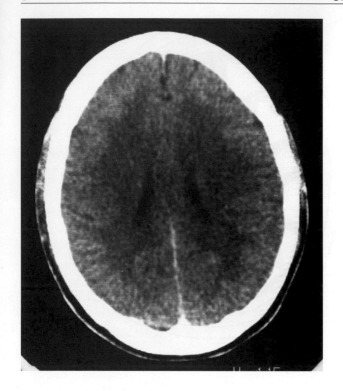

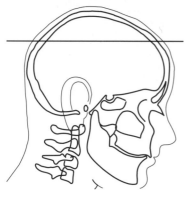

 Frontal lobe
Parietal lobe
Occipital lobe

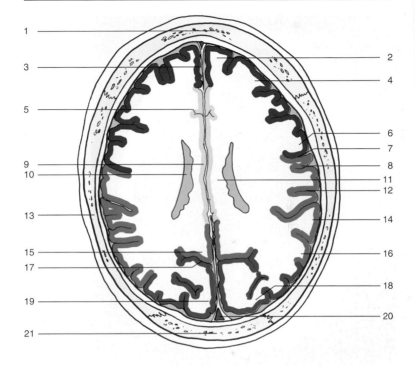

1 Frontal bone
2 Superior frontal gyrus
3 Falx of cerebrum
4 Middle frontal gyrus
5 Cingulate sulcus
6 Precentral gyrus
7 Central sulcus
8 Postcentral gyrus
9 Cingulate gyrus
10 Lateral ventricle
11 Cingulum

12 Postcentral sulcus
13 Parietal bone
14 Supramarginal gyrus
15 Precuneus
16 Angular gyrus
17 Parietooccipital sulcus
18 Occipital gyri
19 Cuneus
20 Superior sagittal sinus
21 Occipital bone

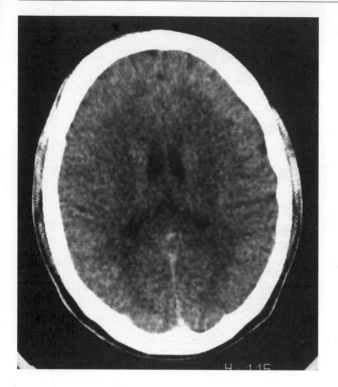

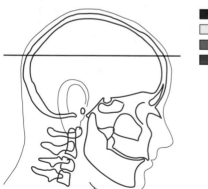

- ■ Frontal lobe
- □ Temporal lobe
- ■ Parietal lobe
- ■ Occipital lobe

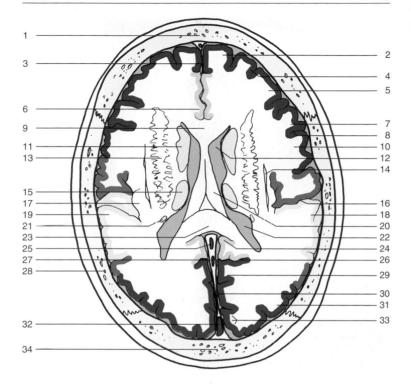

1 Frontal bone
2 Superior frontal gyrus
3 Falx of cerebrum
4 Middle frontal gyrus
5 Middle frontal gyrus
6 Cingulate gyrus
7 Inferior frontal gyrus
8 Precentral sulcus
9 Corpus callosum (body)
10 Precentral gyrus
11 Caudate nucleus (head)
12 Lateral ventricle (anterior horn)
13 Corona radiata
14 Claustrum
15 Thalamus
16 Lateral sulcus
17 Insular lobe
18 Superior temporal gyrus
19 Temporal operculum
20 Fornix
21 Caudate nucleus (tail)
22 Lateral ventricle (collateral trigone,
   choroid plexus)
23 Corpus callosum (splenium)
24 Cingulum
25 Great vein of Galen
26 Parietooccipital sulcus
27 Straight sinus
28 Parietal bone
29 Cuneus
30 Falx of cerebrum
31 Occipital gyri
32 Superior sagittal sinus
33 Striate cortex
34 Occipital bone

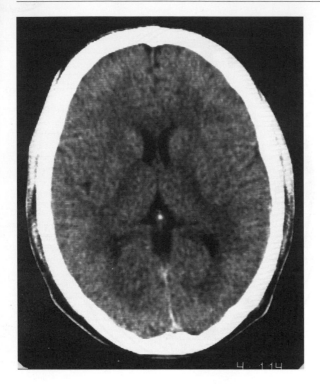

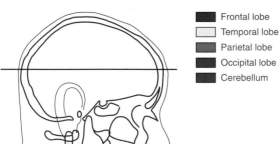

■ Frontal lobe
□ Temporal lobe
■ Parietal lobe
■ Occipital lobe
■ Cerebellum

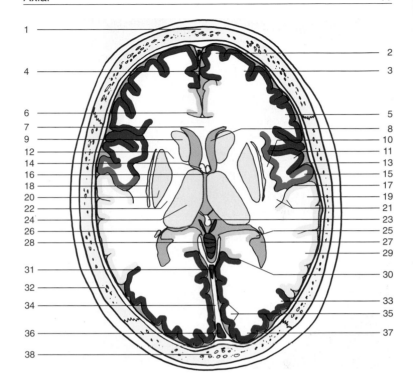

1 Frontal bone
2 Superior frontal gyrus
3 Middle frontal gyrus
4 Falx of cerebrum
5 Inferior frontal gyrus
6 Cingulate gyrus
7 Corpus callosum
8 Lateral ventricle (anterior horn)
9 Caudate nucleus (head)
10 Insular lobe
11 Precentral gyrus
12 Internal capsule (anterior crus)
13 Central sulcus
14 Fornix
15 Postcentral gyrus
16 Interventricular foramen (of Monro)
17 Lateral sulcus
18 Claustrum
19 Superior temporal gyrus
20 Putamen

21 Transverse temporal gyri
   (Heschl's convolutions)
22 Internal capsule (posterior crus)
23 Pineal body
24 Thalamus
25 Hippocampus
26 Caudate nucleus (tail)
27 Lateral ventricle (posterior horn)
28 Vermis of cerebellum
29 Middle temporal gyrus
30 Parietooccipital sulcus
31 Straight sinus
32 Parietal bone
33 Occipital gyri
34 Falx of cerebrum
35 Striate cortex
36 Superior sagittal sinus
37 Occipital pole
38 Occipital bone

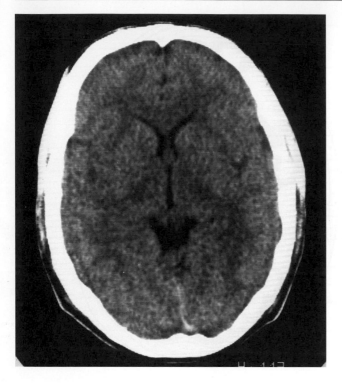

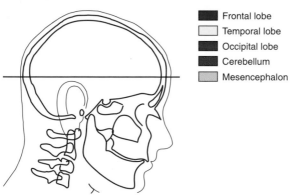

Frontal lobe
Temporal lobe
Occipital lobe
Cerebellum
Mesencephalon

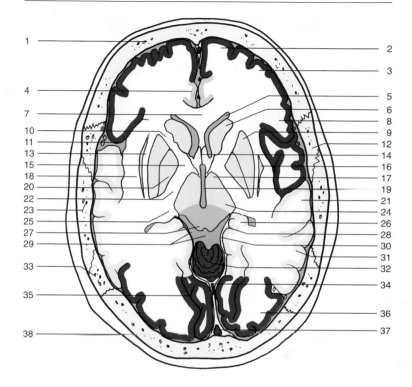

1 Frontal bone
2 Superior frontal gyrus
3 Middle frontal gyrus
4 Cingulate gyrus
5 Lateral ventricle (anterior horn)
6 Caudate nucleus (head)
7 Corpus callosum (genu)
8 Inferior frontal gyrus
9 Putamen
10 Internal capsule (anterior crus)
11 Insular cistern
12 Parietal bone
13 External capsule
14 Precommissural septum
15 Internal capsule (genu)
16 Claustrum
17 Hypothalamus
18 Extreme capsule
19 Third ventricle

20 Globus pallidus
21 Superior temporal gyrus
22 Internal capsule (posterior crus)
23 Temporal bone
24 Thalamus
25 Geniculate body
26 Hippocampus
27 Tectum of mesencephalon (colliculus)
28 Parahippocampal gyrus
29 Quadrigeminal and ambient cisterns
30 Tentorium of cerebellum
31 Middle temporal gyrus
32 Vermis of cerebellum
33 Parietal bone
34 Straight sinus
35 Collateral sulcus
36 Occipital gyri
37 Superior sagittal sinus
38 Occipital bone

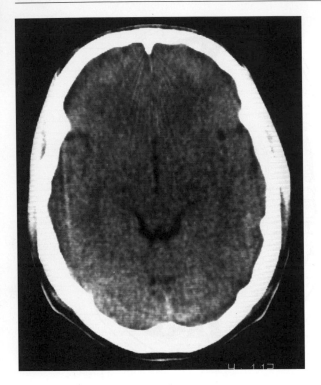

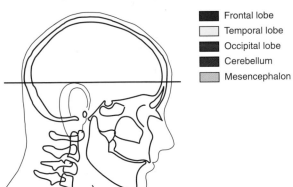

	Frontal lobe
	Temporal lobe
	Occipital lobe
	Cerebellum
	Mesencephalon

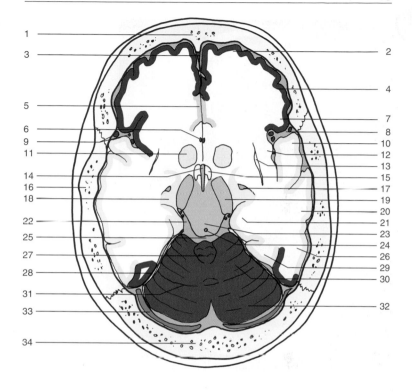

1 Frontal bone
2 Superior frontal gyrus
3 Falx of cerebrum
4 Middle frontal gyrus
5 Cingulate gyrus
6 Anterior cerebral artery
7 Inferior frontal gyrus
8 Lateral sulcus (insular cistern)
9 Insular arteries
10 Superior temporal gyrus
11 Striate body (inferior portion)
12 Insular lobe
13 Claustrum
14 Third ventricle
15 Hypothalamus
16 Parietal bone
17 Lateral ventricle (temporal horn)

18 Uncus
19 Cerebral peduncle
20 Middle temporal gyrus
21 Parahippocampal gyrus
22 Ambient cistern
23 Mesencephalon
24 Cerebral aqueduct
25 Quadrigeminal cistern
26 Inferior temporal gyrus
27 Vermis of cerebellum
28 Tentorium of cerebellum
29 Lateral occipitotemporal gyrus
30 Cerebellum (cranial lobe)
31 Primary fissure
32 Cerebellum (caudal lobe)
33 Transverse sinus
34 Occipital bone

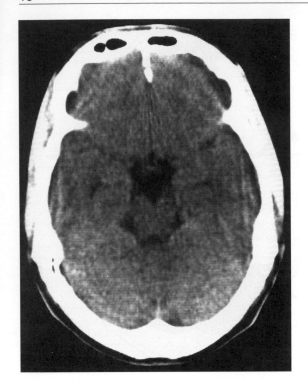

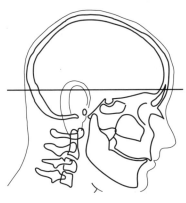

■ Frontal lobe
□ Temporal lobe
■ Cerebellum
■ Mesencephalon
■ Pons

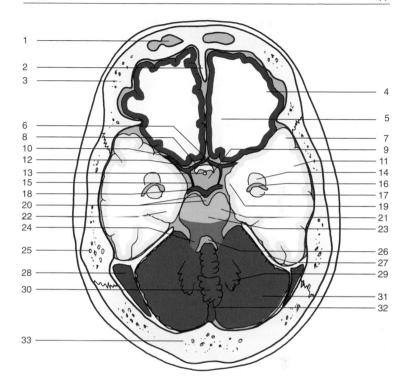

1 Frontal sinus
2 Falx of cerebrum
3 Frontal bone
4 Orbital gyri
5 Straight gyrus
6 Anterior communicating artery
7 Temporal pole
8 Anterior cerebral artery
9 Pentagon of basal cistern
10 Middle cerebral artery
11 Middle temporal gyrus
12 Optic chiasm
13 Infundibulum (pituitary stalk)
14 Amygdaloid body
15 Posterior communicating artery
16 Lateral ventricle (temporal horn)
17 Hippocampus

18 Posterior cerebral artery
19 Uncus
20 Basilar artery and interpeduncular cistern
21 Cerebral peduncle
22 Parahippocampal gyrus
23 Pons
24 Cerebellar peduncle
25 Temporal bone
26 Fourth ventricle
27 Tentorium of cerebellum
28 Sigmoid sinus
29 Dentate nucleus
30 Vermis of cerebellum
31 Cerebellar hemisphere
32 Occipital sinus
33 Occipital bone

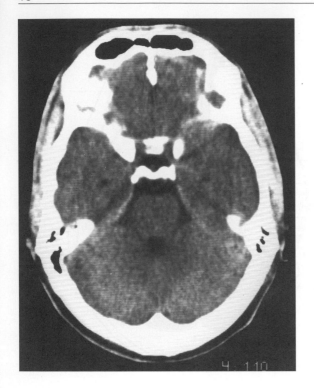

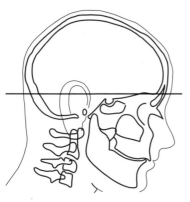

■ Frontal lobe
□ Temporal lobe
■ Cerebellum
■ Pons

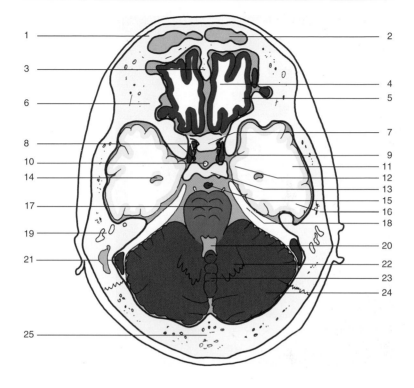

1 Frontal bone
2 Frontal sinus
3 Crista galli
4 Straight gyrus
5 Orbital gyri
6 Sphenoid bone
7 Anterior clinoid process
8 Cavernous sinus
9 Internal carotid artery
10 Infundibulum (pituitary stalk)
11 Middle temporal gyrus
12 Parahippocampal gyrus
13 Clivus
14 Lateral ventricle (temporal horn)
15 Basilar artery
16 Inferior temporal gyrus
17 Pons
18 Tentorium of cerebellum
19 Temporal bone
20 Fourth ventricle
21 Sigmoid sinus
22 Dentate nucleus
23 Vermis of cerebellum
24 Cerebellar hemisphere
25 Occipital bone

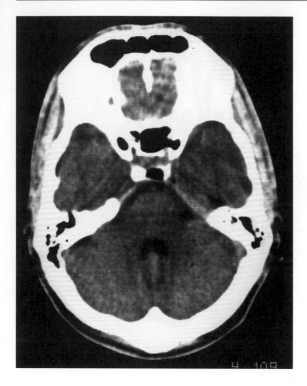

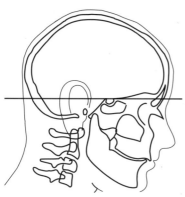

 Frontal lobe
 Temporal lobe
Cerebellum
Pons

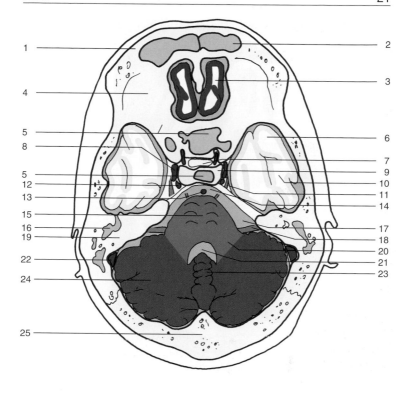

1 Frontal bone
2 Frontal sinus
3 Straight gyrus
4 Sphenoid bone (lesser wing)
   and orbital roof
5 Sphenoid sinus
6 Temporal pole
7 Pituitary gland
8 Internal carotid artery
9 Dorsum sellae
10 Inferior temporal gyrus
11 Trigeminal nerve
12 Cavernous sinus

13 Basilar artery
14 Prepontine cistern
15 Pons
16 Mastoid antrum
17 Cerebellopontine angle cistern
18 Facial and vestibulocochlear nerves
19 Temporal bone (petrous part)
20 Middle cerebellar peduncle
21 Fourth ventricle (with plexus)
22 Sigmoid sinus
23 Vermis of cerebellum
24 Cerebellum (caudal lobe)
25 Occipital bone

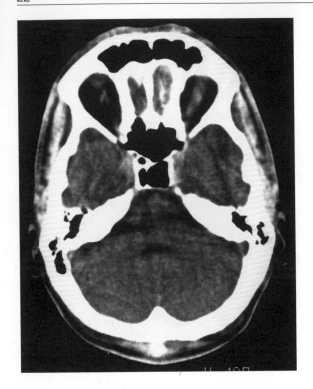

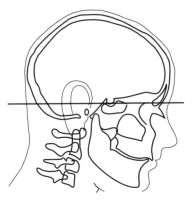

■ Frontal lobe
□ Temporal lobe
■ Cerebellum
■ Pons

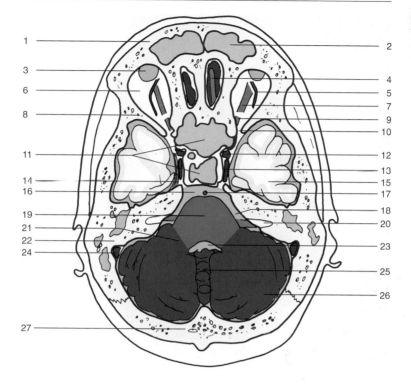

1 Frontal bone
2 Frontal sinus
3 Ocular bulb
4 Straight gyrus
5 Ophthalmic vein, olfactory bulb
6 Orbit
7 Superior rectus muscle
8 Sphenoid bone
9 Optic nerve
10 Superior orbital fissure
11 Sphenoid sinus
12 Cavernous sinus
13 Internal carotid artery
14 Trigeminal nerve

15 Inferior temporal gyrus
16 Prepontine cistern
17 Basilar artery
18 Cerebellopontine angle cistern
19 Pons
20 Internal auditory canal
21 Middle and inferior cerebellar
   peduncles
22 Temporal bone (petrous part)
23 Fourth ventricle
24 Sigmoid sinus
25 Vermis of cerebellum
26 Cerebellum (caudal lobe)
27 Occipital bone

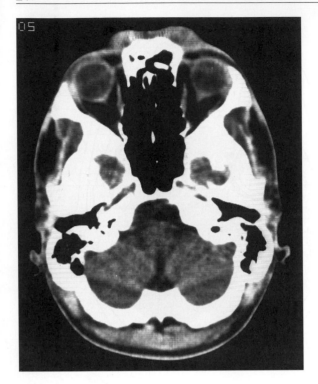

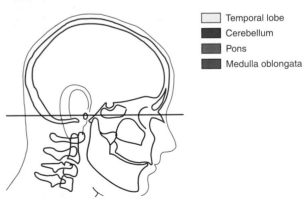

Temporal lobe
Cerebellum
Pons
Medulla oblongata

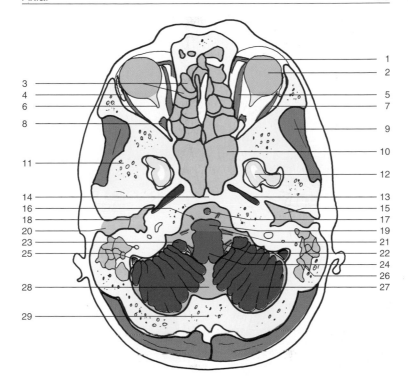

1 Superior oblique muscle
2 Ocular bulb
3 Ethmoid labyrinth
4 Lacrimal gland
5 Medial rectus muscle
6 Optic nerve
7 Lateral rectus muscle
8 Superior rectus muscle
9 Temporal muscle
10 Sphenoid sinus
11 Temporal bone
12 Temporal lobe (base)
13 Internal carotid artery
14 Clivus
15 Tympanic cavity

16 Abducens nerve
17 Basilar artery
18 Tympanic membrane
19 Pons
20 External auditory canal
21 Anterior inferior cerebellar artery
22 Glossopharyngeal and vagus nerves
23 Floccule
24 Medulla oblongata
25 Sigmoid sinus
26 Mastoid air cells
27 Cerebellar hemisphere (caudal lobe)
28 Cerebellomedullary cistern
29 Occipital bone

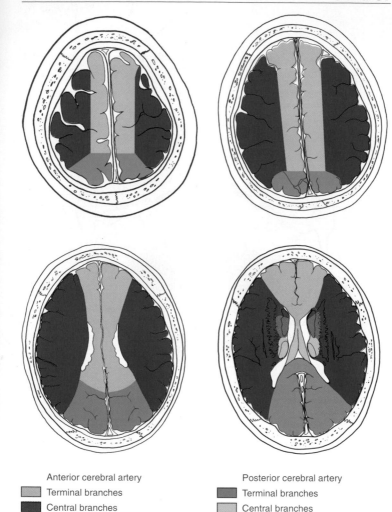

Anterior cerebral artery

Terminal branches

Central branches

Middle cerebral artery

Terminal branches

central branches

Posterior cerebral artery

Terminal branches

Central branches

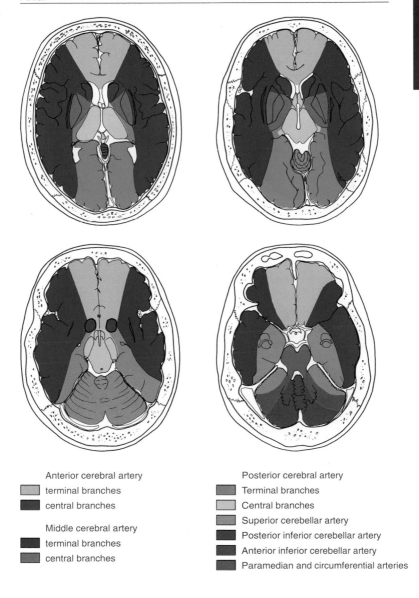

Anterior cerebral artery
- terminal branches
- central branches

Middle cerebral artery
- terminal branches
- central branches

Posterior cerebral artery
- Terminal branches
- Central branches
- Superior cerebellar artery
- Posterior inferior cerebellar artery
- Anterior inferior cerebellar artery
- Paramedian and circumferential arteries

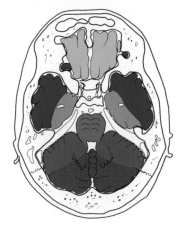
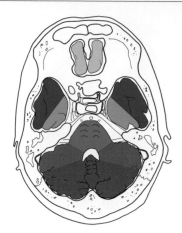
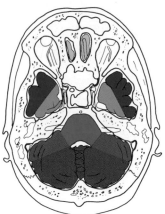

Anterior cerebral artery
- Terminal branches
- Central branches

Middle cerebral artery
- Terminal branches
- Central branches

Posterior cerebral artery
- Terminal branches
- Central branches
- Superior cerebellar artery
- Posterior inferior cerebellar artery
- Anterior inferior cerebellar artery
- Paramedian and curcumferential arteries

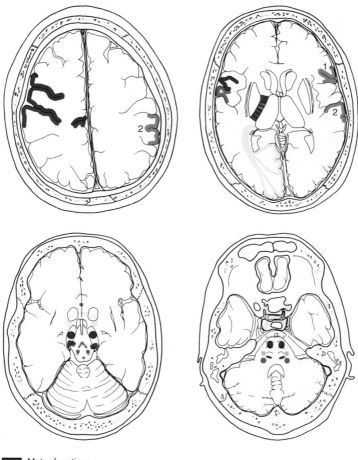

Motor functions

Sensory functions
Medial lemniscus tract
Spinothalamic tract
Mesencephalic nucleus of trigeminal nerve

Oculomotor nucleus and tract
Optic tract
Speech area (1=motor, 2=sensory)

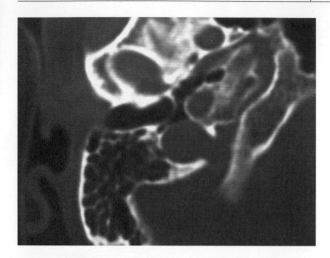

1

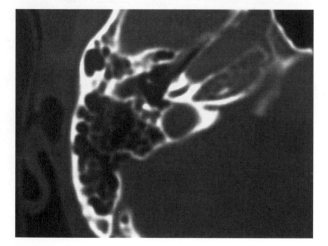

2

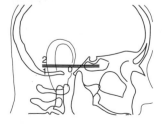

frontal

lateral ☐ medial

occipital

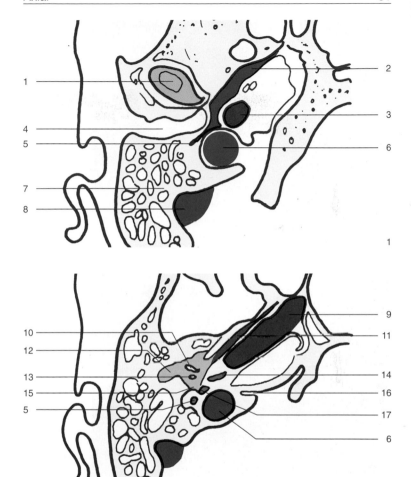

1 Temporomandibular joint
  (mandibular fossa and articular disk)
2 Auditory (eustachian) tube
3 Internal carotid artery
4 External auditory canal
5 Facial canal
6 Internal jugular vein
7 Mastoid process
8 Sigmoid sinus

9 Carotid canal
10 Malleus (handle)
11 Tensor muscle of tympanum (canal)
12 Middle ear
13 Incus (long crus)
14 Cochlea (base)
15 Tympanic sinus
16 Vestibular aqueduct
17 Round window

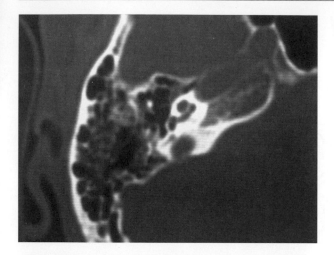

3

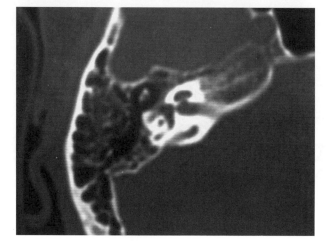

4

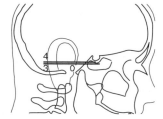

frontal

lateral ▢ medial

occipital

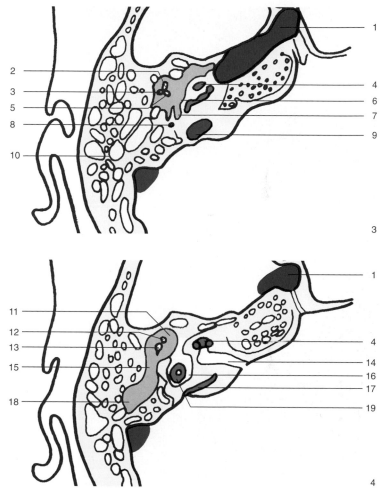

1 Internal carotid artery (canal)
2 Malleus (handle)
3 Incus (long crus)
4 Cochlea
5 Stapes
6 Oval window
7 Tympanic sinus
8 Facial canal
9 Internal jugular vein (bulb)
10 Mastoid air cells

11 Epitympanic recess
12 Malleus (head)
13 Incus (short crus)
14 Internal auditory canal
15 Aditus ad antrum
16 Vestibule
17 Posterior semicircular canal
18 Mastoid antrum
19 Lateral semicircular canal

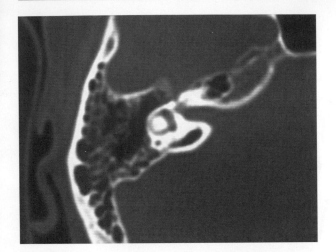

5

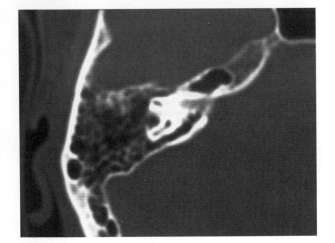

6

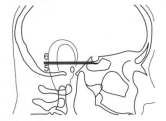

frontal

lateral   ☐   medial

occipital

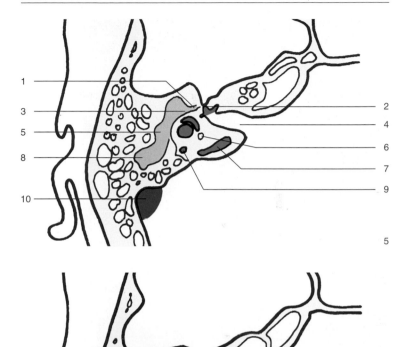

5

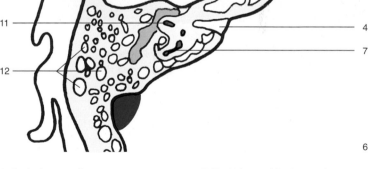

6

1 Geniculate ganglion
2 Facial nerve (first part)
3 Facial nerve (second part)
4 Internal auditory canal
5 Tympanic cavity
6 Vestibule

7 Posterior semicircular canal
8 Mastoid antrum
9 Lateral semicircular canal
10 Sigmoid sinus
11 Anterior semicircular canal
12 Mastoid air cells

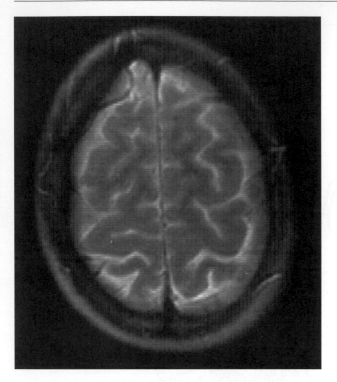

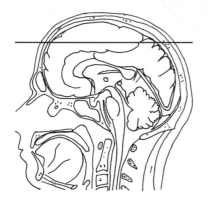

■ Frontal lobe
■ Parietal lobe

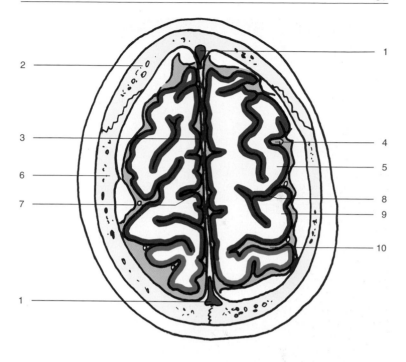

1 Superior sagittal sinus
2 Frontal bone
3 Falx of cerebrum
4 Precentral sulcus
5 Precentral gyrus

6 Parietal bone
7 Longitudinal fissure
8 Central sulcus
9 Postcentral gyrus
10 Postcentral sulcus

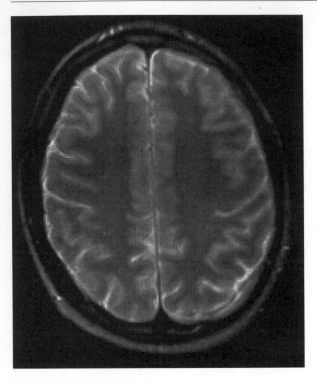

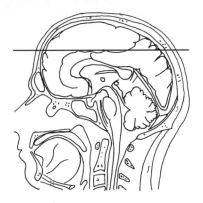

■ Frontal lobe
■ Parietal lobe

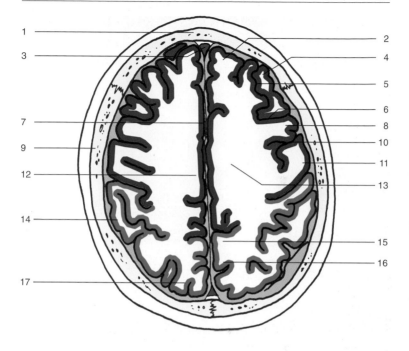

1 Frontal bone
2 Superior frontal gyrus
3 Superior sagittal sinus
4 Middle frontal gyrus
5 Superior frontal sulcus
6 Precentral sulcus
7 Falx of cerebrum
8 Precentral gyrus
9 Parietal bone

10 Central sulcus
11 Postcentral gyrus
12 Paracentral lobule
13 Semioval center
14 Parietal lobule
15 Paracentral lobule
16 Precuneus
17 Parietooccipital sulcus

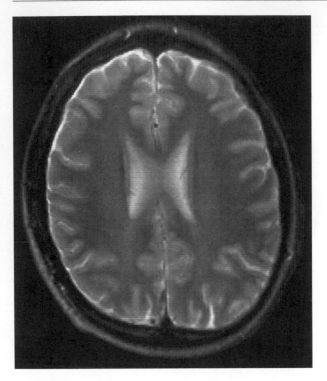

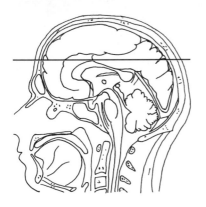

Frontal lobe
Parietal lobe
Occipital lobe

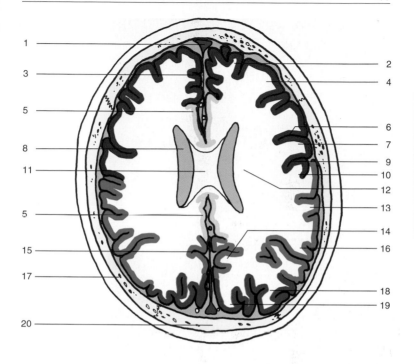

1 Superior sagittal sinus
2 Superior frontal gyrus
3 Falx of cerebrum
4 Middle frontal gyrus
5 Cingulum
6 Precentral sulcus
7 Precentral gyrus
8 Lateral ventricle
9 Central sulcus
10 Postcentral gyrus
11 Corpus callosum
12 Corona radiata
13 Supramarginal gyrus
14 Precuneus
15 Parietooccipital sulcus
16 Angular gyrus
17 Parietal bone
18 Occipital gyri
19 Cuneus
20 Occipital bone

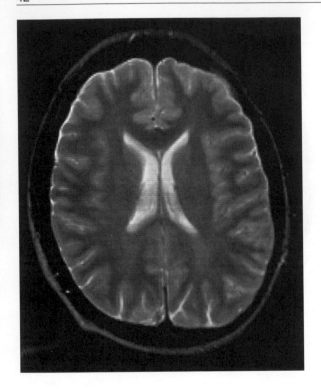

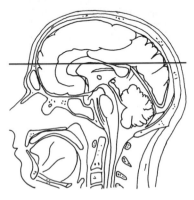

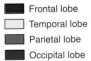

Frontal lobe
Temporal lobe
Parietal lobe
Occipital lobe

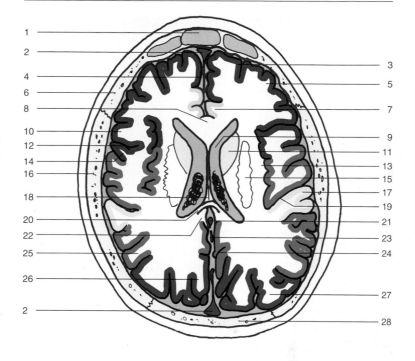

1 Frontal sinus
2 Superior sagittal sinus
3 Superior frontal gyrus
4 Falx of cerebrum
5 Middle frontal gyrus
6 Frontal bone
7 Cingulate gyrus
8 Corpus callosum
9 Lateral ventricle (anterior horn)
10 Precentral gyrus
11 Caudate nucleus (head)
12 Central sulcus
13 Insular lobe
14 Postcentral gyrus

15 Corona radiata
16 Parietal bone
17 Superior temporal gyrus
18 Fornix (body)
19 Lateral sulcus
20 Corpus callosum (splenium)
21 Great vein of Galen
22 Cingulate gyrus
23 Straight sinus
24 Parietooccipital sulcus
25 Angular gyrus
26 Cuneus
27 Occipital gyri
28 Occipital bone

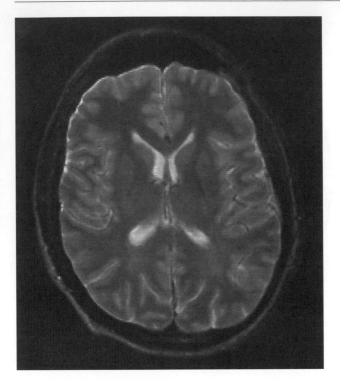

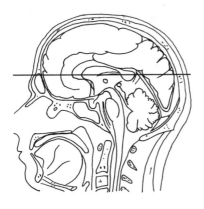

Frontal lobe
Temporal lobe
Parietal lobe
Occipital lobe

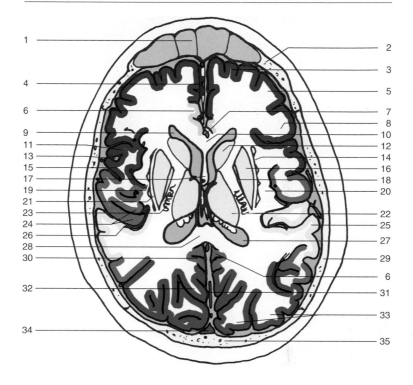

1 Frontal sinus
2 Frontal bone
3 Superior frontal gyrus
4 Falx of cerebrum (interhemispheric fissure)
5 Middle frontal gyrus
6 Cingulate gyrus
7 Pericallosal artery
8 Inferior frontal gyrus
9 Lateral ventricle (anterior horn)
10 Corpus callosum (genu)
11 Precentral gyrus
12 Caudate nucleus (head)
13 Central sulcus
14 Claustrum
15 Postcentral gyrus
16 Putamen
17 Pellucid septum
18 Globus pallidus

19 Extreme capsule
20 Insular lobe
21 External capsule
22 Thalamus
23 Internal capsule
24 Transverse temporal gyri
   (Heschl's convolutions)
25 Superior temporal gyrus
26 Lateral sulcus
27 Lateral ventricle (posterior horn)
28 Corpus callosum (splenium)
29 Parietal bone
30 Parietooccipital sulcus
31 Straight sinus
32 Cuneus
33 Occipital gyri
34 Superior sagittal sinus
35 Occipital bone

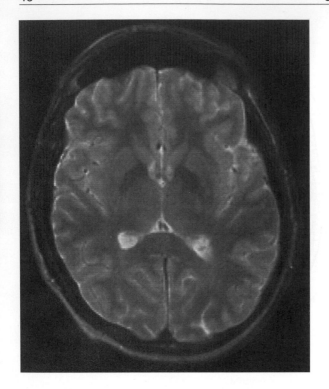

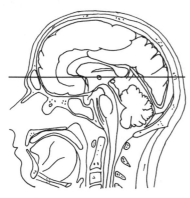

Frontal lobe
Temporal lobe
Parietal lobe
Occipital lobe

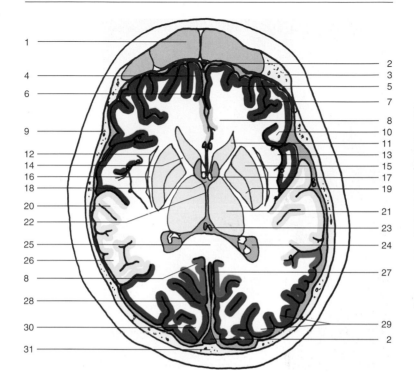

1 Frontal sinus
2 Superior sagittal sinus
3 Frontal bone
4 Frontal pole
5 Superior frontal gyrus
6 Falx of cerebrum and interhemispheric fissure
7 Middle frontal gyrus
8 Cingulate gyrus
9 Parietal bone
10 Frontal operculum
11 Caudate nucleus (head)
12 Claustrum
13 Insular lobe
14 Internal capsule
15 Putamen
16 External capsule
17 Fornix (anterior column)
18 Interventricular foramen (of Monro)
19 Globus pallidus
20 Superior temporal gyrus
21 Thalamus
22 Third ventricle
23 Posterior choroid artery
24 Lateral ventricle (posterior horn)
25 Corpus callosum (splenium)
26 Middle temporal gyrus
27 Straight sinus
28 Calcarine sulcus
29 Occipital gyri
30 Occipital pole
31 Occipital bone

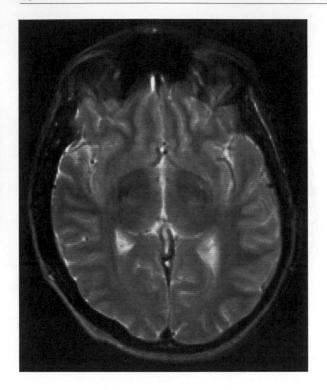

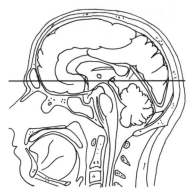

Frontal lobe
Temporal lobe
Occipital lobe

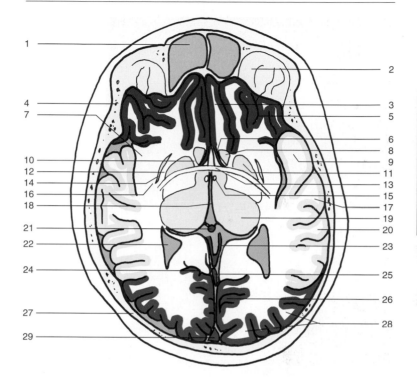

1 Frontal sinus
2 Orbital roof
3 Straight gyrus
4 Frontal bone
5 Inferior frontal gyrus
6 Anterior cerebral artery
7 Insular lobe
8 Caudate nucleus (head)
9 Superior temporal gyrus
10 Internal capsule
11 Putamen
12 External capsule
13 Anterior commissure
14 Claustrum
15 Fornix (postcommissural)

16 Extreme capsule
17 Middle temporal gyrus
18 Third ventricle
19 Thalamus
20 Inferior temporal gyrus
21 Pineal body
22 Lateral ventricle (posterior horn)
23 Internal cerebral vein
24 Parietooccipital sulcus
25 Great vein of Galen
26 Striate cortex
27 Occipital bone
28 Occipital gyri
29 Superior sagittal sinus

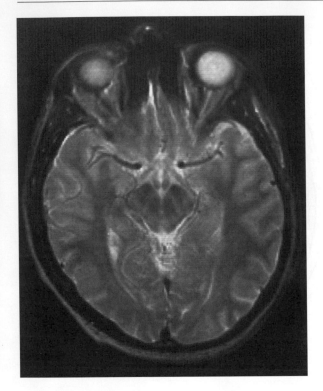

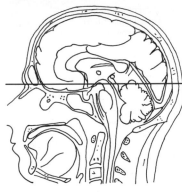

 Frontal lobe
Temporal lobe
 Occipital lobe
Cerebellum
Mesencephalon

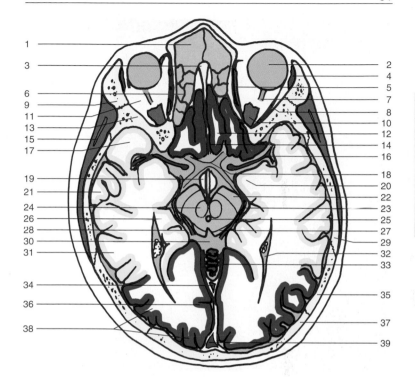

1 Frontal sinus
2 Ocular bulb
3 Crista galli
4 Lacrimal gland
5 Superior oblique muscle
6 Ethmoid labyrinth
7 Optic nerve
8 Lateral rectus muscle
9 Zygomatic bone
10 Superior rectus muscle
11 Orbit
12 Straight gyrus
13 Sphenoid bone
14 Anterior cerebral artery
15 Temporal muscle
16 Middle cerebral artery
17 Superior temporal gyrus
18 Optic chiasm
19 Hypothalamus
20 Uncus

21 Middle temporal gyrus
22 Cerebral peduncle
23 Posterior cerebral artery
24 Red nucleus
25 Aqueduct
26 Hippocampus
27 Cranial colliculus
28 Ambient cistern
29 Temporal bone
30 Bichat's canal (cisterna venae
    magnae cerebri)
31 Inferior temporal gyrus
32 Lateral ventricle (temporal horn)
33 Cranial lobe of cerebellum
34 Straight sinus
35 Parietal bone
36 Calcarine sulcus
37 Occipital bone
38 Superior sagittal sinus

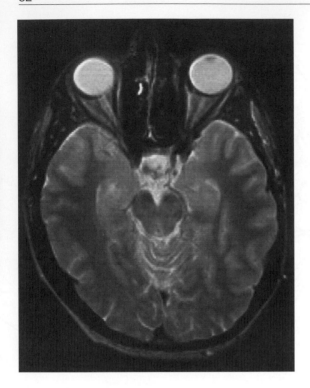

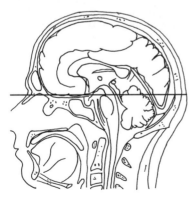

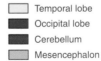

Temporal lobe

Occipital lobe

Cerebellum

Mesencephalon

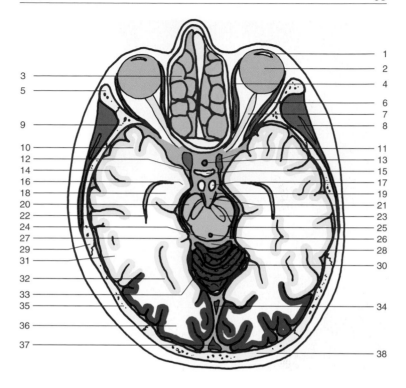

1 Lens
2 Ocular bulb
3 Ethmoid labyrinth
4 Medial rectus muscle
5 Zygomatic bone
6 Lateral rectus muscle
7 Optic nerve
8 Temporal muscle
9 Sphenoid bone
10 Superior temporal gyrus
11 Internal carotid artery
12 Posterior communicating artery
13 Infundibulum
14 Middle temporal gyrus
15 Dorsum sellae
16 Uncus
17 Mammillary body
18 Hippocampus
19 Oculomotor nerve

20 Cerebral peduncle
21 Interpeduncular cistern
22 Lateral ventricle (temporal horn)
23 Black substance
24 Caudal colliculus
25 Posterior cerebral artery (in ambient cistern)
26 Aqueduct
27 Parahippocampal gyrus
28 Ambient cistern
29 Temporal bone
30 Cranial lobe of cerebellum
31 Inferior temporal gyrus
32 Collateral sulcus
33 Tentorium of cerebellum
34 Straight sinus
35 Parietal bone
36 Occipital gyri
37 Superior sagittal sinus
38 Occipital bone

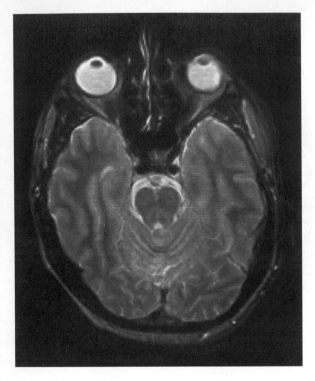

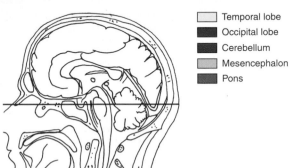

- ☐ Temporal lobe
- ■ Occipital lobe
- ■ Cerebellum
- ▨ Mesencephalon
- ■ Pons

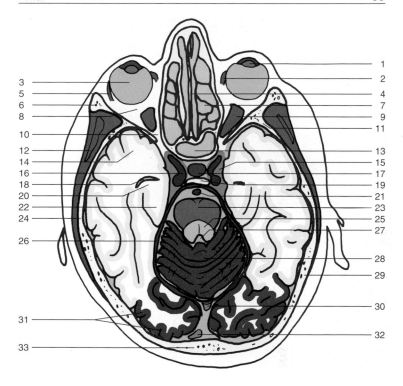

1 Lens
2 Medial rectus muscle
3 Ocular bulb
4 Nasal septum
5 Lateral rectus muscle
6 Zygomatic bone
7 Ethmoid labyrinth
8 Orbit
9 Inferior rectus muscle
10 Superior orbital fissure
11 Sphenoid bone
12 Temporal muscle
13 Sphenoid sinus
14 Temporal lobe
15 Cavernous sinus
16 Internal carotid artery
17 Pituitary gland

18 Lateral ventricle (temporal horn)
19 Dorsum sellae
20 Hippocampus
21 Basilar artery
22 Parahippocampal gyrus
23 Pons
24 Temporal bone
25 Reticular formation
26 Tentorium of cerebellum
27 Fourth ventricle
28 Cranial lobe of cerebellum
29 Parietal bone
30 Straight sinus
31 Occipital gyri
32 Superior sagittal sinus
33 Occipital bone

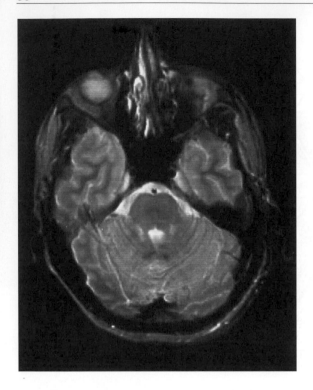

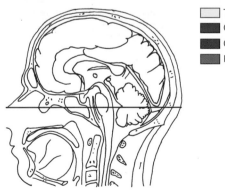

Temporal lobe
Occipital lobe
Cerebellum
Pons

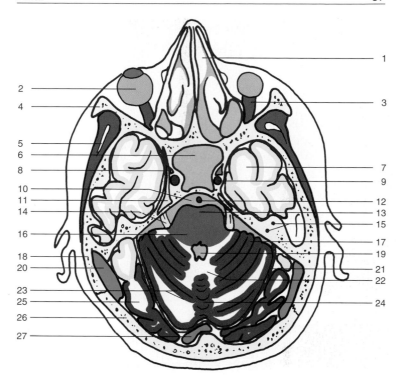

1 Nasal cavity
2 Ocular bulb
3 Inferior rectus muscle
4 Zygomatic bone
5 Temporal muscle
6 Sphenoid sinus
7 Temporal lobe
8 Cavernous sinus
9 Internal carotid artery
10 Cerebellopontine angle cistern
11 Trigeminal (gasserian) ganglion in
   Trigeminal (Meckel's) cave
12 Basilar artery
13 Pons

14 Trigeminal nerve (CN V)
15 Anterior semicircular canal
16 Middle cerebellar peduncle
17 Cerebellum (cranial lobe)
18 Temporal bone
19 Fourth ventricle
20 Transverse sinus
21 Tentorium of cerebellum
22 Dentate nucleus
23 Cerebellum (caudal lobe)
24 Nodule of vermis
25 Occipital pole
26 Occipital bone
27 Confluence of sinuses

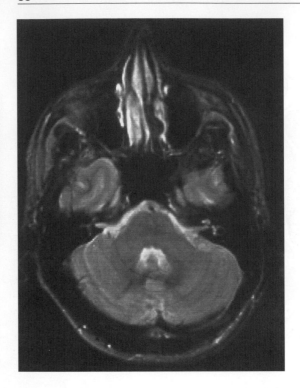

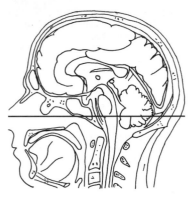

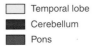

☐ Temporal lobe
■ Cerebellum
■ Pons

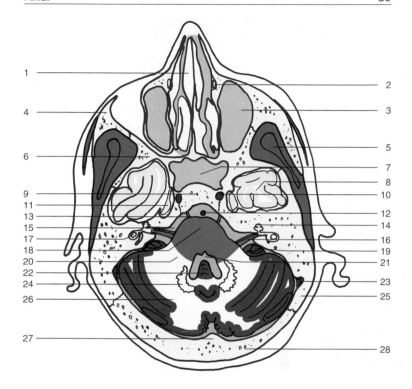

1 Nasal septum
2 Nasolacrimal duct
3 Maxillary sinus
4 Zygomatic bone
5 Temporal muscle
6 Sphenoid bone
7 Sphenoid sinus
8 Temporal lobe (base)
9 Clivus
10 Internal carotid artery
11 Trigeminal ganglion
12 Basilar artery
13 Abducens nerve
14 Cochlea

15 Cerebellopontine angle cistern
16 Vestibulocochlear nerve (CN VIII)
17 Semicircular canal
18 Pons
19 Floccule
20 Middle cerebellar peduncle
21 Fourth ventricle
22 Nodule of vermis
23 Sigmoid sinus
24 Dentate nucleus
25 Temporal bone
26 Cerebellum (caudal lobe)
27 Internal occipital protuberance
28 Occipital bone

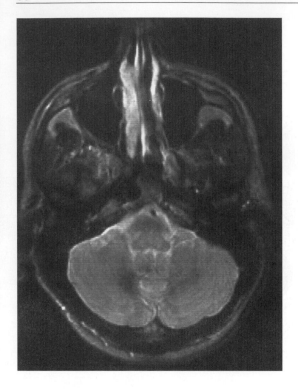

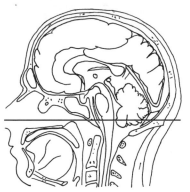

■ Cerebellum
■ Pons
■ Medulla oblongata

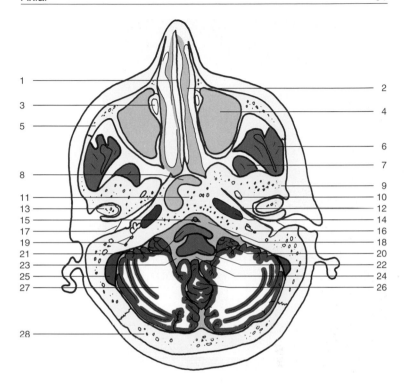

1 Nasal septum
2 Nasal cavity
3 Nasolacrimal duct
4 Maxillary sinus
5 Zygomatic bone
6 Temporal muscle
7 Lateral pterygoid muscle
8 Sphenoid sinus
9 Temporal bone
10 Mandibular nerve
    (third branch of trigeminal nerve)
11 Clivus
12 Auditory tube
13 Temporomandibular joint
14 Internal carotid artery

15 Basilar artery
16 Cochlea
17 External auditory canal
18 Prepontine cistern
19 Posterior semicircular canal
20 Floccule
21 Pons
22 Medulla oblongata
23 Lateral aperture of fourth ventricle
    (Luschka's foramen)
24 Fourth ventricle
25 Sigmoid sinus
26 Uvula vermis
27 Cerebellum (caudal lobe)
28 Occipital bone

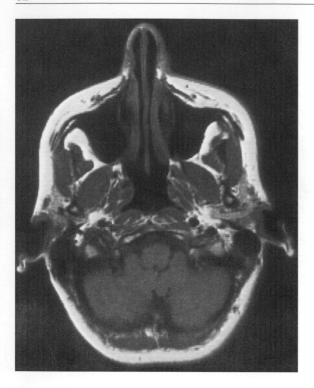

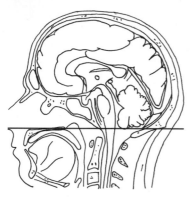

■ Cerebellum
■ Medulla oblongata

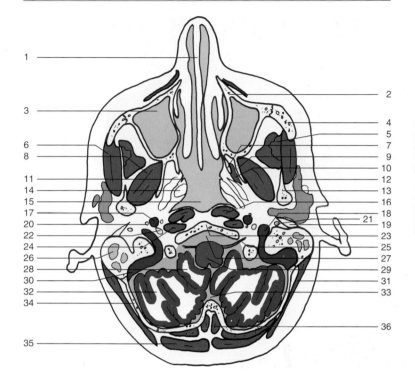

1 Nasal septum
2 Maxillary bone
3 Maxillary sinus
4 Zygomatic bone
5 Temporal muscle
6 Masseter muscle
7 Medial pterygoid plate
8 Lateral pterygoid muscle
9 Lateral pterygoid plate
10 Medial pterygoid muscle and tensor
   veli palatini muscle
11 Pharyngeal ostium of auditory tube
12 Parotid gland
13 Condyle of mandible
14 Auditory tube
15 Nasopharynx
16 Longus capitis muscle
17 Internal carotid artery
18 Internal jugular vein (bulb)
19 Styloid process

20 Glossopharyngeal nerve
21 Facial nerve (CN VII)
22 Vagus nerve (CN X)
23 Clivus
24 Rectus capitis anterior muscle
25 Hypoglossal nerve (CN XII)
26 Mastoid process
27 Posterior basal cistern
28 Cerebellar tonsil
29 Medulla oblongata (with central canal)
30 Sigmoid sinus
31 Splenius capitis muscle
32 Cerebellum (caudal, posterior lobe)
33 Cerebellomedullary cistern
34 Occipital bone
35 Semispinalis capitis muscle
36 Rectus capitis posterior muscles
   (minor and major)

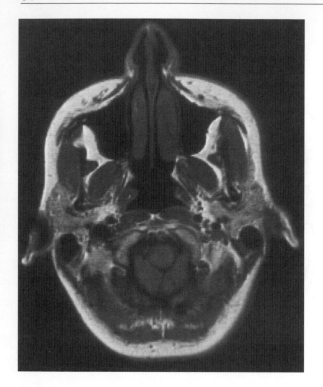

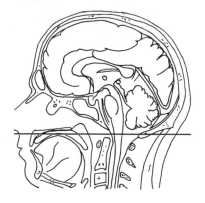

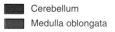 Cerebellum

Medulla oblongata

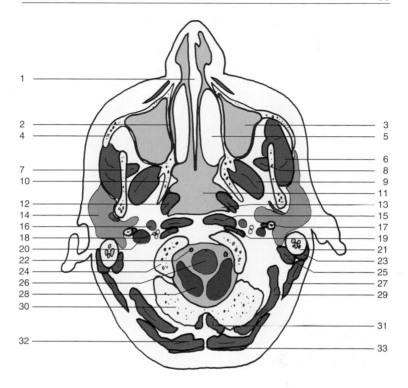

1 Nasal septum
2 Medial wall of maxillary sinus
3 Maxillary sinus
4 Zygomatic bone (arch)
5 Nasal conchae
6 Masseter muscle
7 Mandible
8 Temporal muscle
9 Lateral pterygoid muscle
10 Pterygoid process
11 Nasopharynx
12 Auditory tube
13 Lateral pharyngeal (Rosenmüller's) recess
14 Parotid gland
15 Longus capitis muscle
16 Internal carotid artery
17 Styloid process and styloid muscles
18 Vagus, accessory, and hypoglossal nerves
19 Rectus capitis anterior muscle
20 Internal jugular vein
21 Mastoid process
22 Vertebral artery
23 Sternocleidomastoid muscle
24 Occipital condyle
25 Digastric muscle (posterior belly)
26 Medulla oblongata
27 Splenius capitis muscle
28 Cerebellar tonsil
29 Rectus capitis posterior muscle (major)
30 Occipital bone
31 Rectus capitis posterior muscle (minor)
32 Semispinalis capitis muscle
33 Trapezius muscle

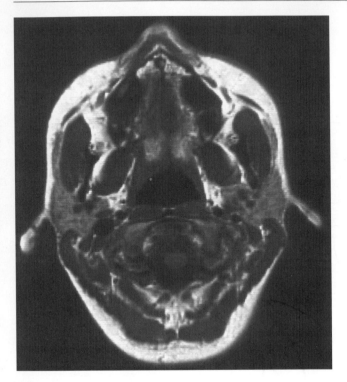

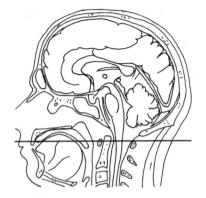

Cerebellum

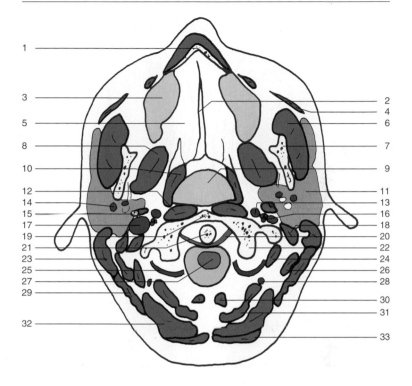

1 Incisive bone
3 Maxillary sinus
5 Palatine process
8 Medial pterygoid muscle
10 Levator veli palatini muscle
12 Longus capitis muscle
14 Retromandibular vein
15 Styloid process
17 Internal jugular vein
19 Atlas (anterior arch)
21 Odontoid process of axis
23 Sternocleidomastoid muscle
25 Vertebral artery
27 Spinal cord
29 Splenius capitis muscle
32 Semispinalis capitis muscle

1 Incisive bone
2 Nasal crest
3 Maxillary sinus
4 Zygomatic muscle
5 Palatine process
6 Masseter muscle
7 Mandible (ramus)
8 Medial pterygoid muscle
9 Nasopharynx
10 Levator veli palatini muscle
11 Parotid gland
12 Longus capitis muscle
13 Internal carotid artery
14 Retromandibular vein
15 Styloid process
16 Vagus, accessory, and hypoglossal nerves
17 Internal jugular vein
18 Digastric muscle (posterior belly)
19 Atlas (anterior arch)
20 Cruciform ligament of atlas
21 Odontoid process of axis
22 Atlas (lateral mass)
23 Sternocleidomastoid muscle
24 Inferior oblique muscle
25 Vertebral artery
26 Longissimus capitis muscle
27 Spinal cord
28 Deep cervical vein
29 Splenius capitis muscle
30 Rectus capitis posterior muscle (minor)
31 Rectus capitis posterior muscle (major)
32 Semispinalis capitis muscle
33 Trapezius muscle

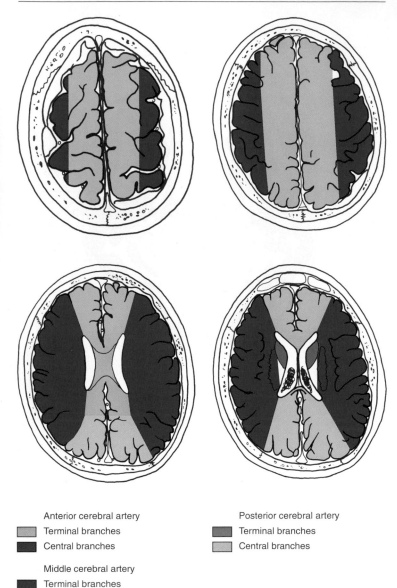

Anterior cerebral artery
Terminal branches
Central branches

Middle cerebral artery
Terminal branches
Central branches

Posterior cerebral artery
Terminal branches
Central branches

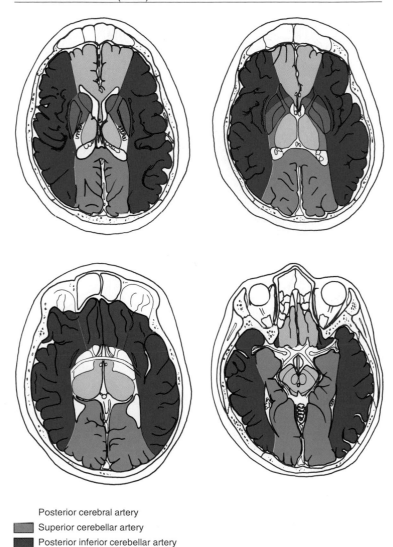

Posterior cerebral artery
Superior cerebellar artery
Posterior inferior cerebellar artery
Anterior inferior cerebellar artery
Paramedian and circumferential arteries

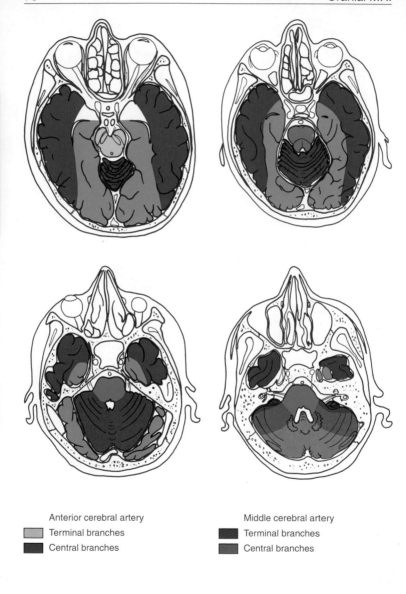

Anterior cerebral artery
Terminal branches
Central branches

Middle cerebral artery
Terminal branches
Central branches

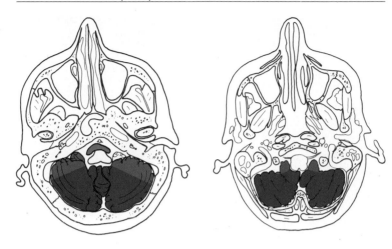

Anterior cerebral artery
▮ Terminal branches
▯ Central branches

Posterior cerebral artery
▮ Superior cerebellar artery
▮ Posterior inferior cerebellar artery
▮ Anterior inferior cerebellar artery
▮ Paramedian and circumferential arteries

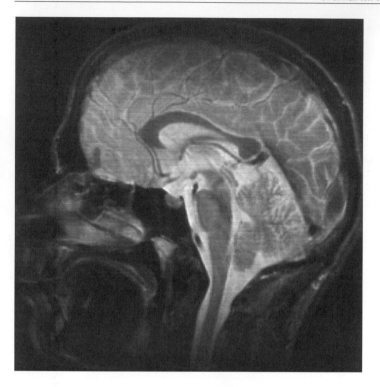

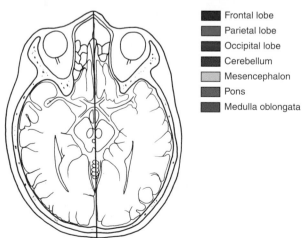

- Frontal lobe
- Parietal lobe
- Occipital lobe
- Cerebellum
- Mesencephalon
- Pons
- Medulla oblongata

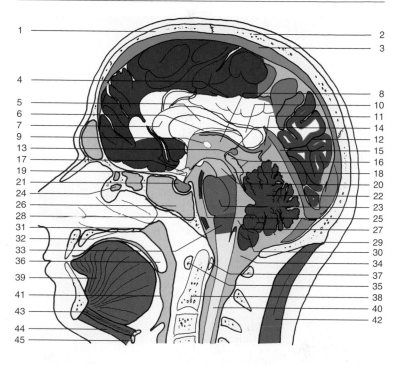

1   Frontal bone
2   Parietal bone
3   Superior sagittal sinus
4   Cingulate sulcus
5   Pellucid septum
6   Internal cerebral vein
7   Corpus callosum (genu)
8   Third ventricle
9   Intermediate mass
10 Corpus callosum (splenium)
11 Great vein of Galen
12 Parietooccipital sulcus
13 Anterior and posterior commissures
14 Pineal body
15 Straight sinus
16 Cranial and caudal colliculi
17 Optic nerve
18 Aqueduct
19 Infundibulum
20 Mesencephalic tegmentum
21 Pituitary gland
22 Cerebellum
23 Pons

24 Ethmoid labyrinth
25 Basilar artery
26 Sphenoid sinus
27 Fourth ventricle
28 Clivus
29 Occipital bone
      (external occipital protuberance)
30 Uvula vermis
31 Nasopharynx
32 Hard palate
33 Medulla oblongata
34 Cerebellomedullary cistern
35 Atlas (arch)
36 Uvula
37 Transverse ligament of atlas
38 Odontoid process of axis
39 Genioglossus muscle
40 Spinal cord
41 Oropharynx
42 Semispinalis capitis muscle
43 Geniohyoid muscle
44 Mylohyoid muscle
45 Hyoid bone

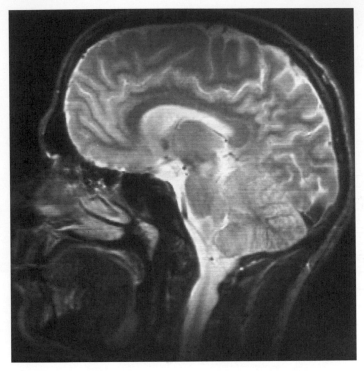

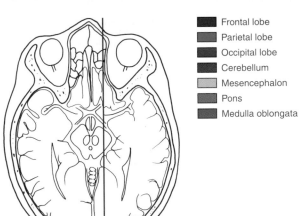

■ Frontal lobe
■ Parietal lobe
■ Occipital lobe
■ Cerebellum
■ Mesencephalon
■ Pons
■ Medulla oblongata

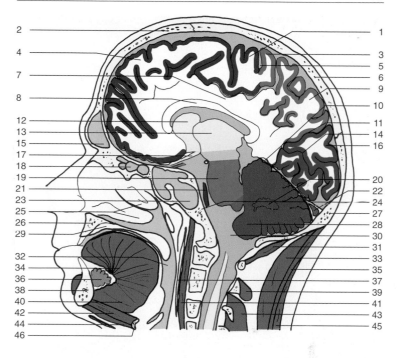

1 Precentral gyrus
2 Frontal bone
3 Postcentral gyrus
4 Superior frontal gyrus
5 Central sulcus
6 Parietal bone
7 Cingulum
8 Corpus callosum (body)
9 Precuneus
10 Tentorium of cerebellum
11 Parietooccipital sulcus
12 Caudate nucleus
13 Thalamus
14 Calcarine sulcus
15 Frontal sinus
16 Occipital gyri
17 Optic nerve
18 Ethmoid labyrinth
19 Pons
20 Dentate nucleus
21 Basilar artery
22 Transverse sinus
23 Sphenoid sinus
24 Clivus

25 Middle and inferior nasal conchae
26 Maxilla
27 Occipital bone
28 Cerebellar tonsil
29 Hard palate
30 Cerebellomedullary cistern
31 Rectus capitis posterior muscle (minor)
32 Oropharynx
33 Semispinalis capitis muscle
34 Genioglossus muscle
35 Splenius capitis muscle
36 Sublingual gland
37 Constrictor muscle of pharynx
38 Mandible (body)
39 Rectus capitis posterior muscle
40 Hyoglossus muscle
41 Longus capitis muscle
42 Geniohyoid muscle
43 Semispinalis cervicis muscle
44 Mylohyoid muscle
45 Trapezius muscle
46 Hyoid bone

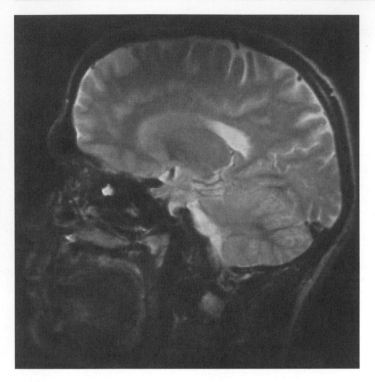

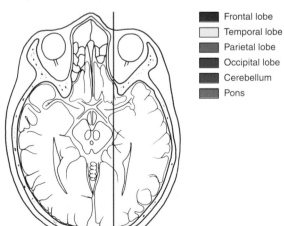

■ Frontal lobe
☐ Temporal lobe
■ Parietal lobe
■ Occipital lobe
■ Cerebellum
■ Pons

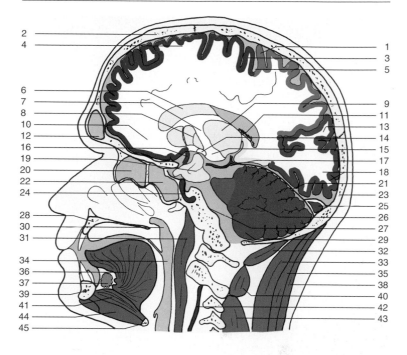

1 Postcentral gyrus
2 Frontal bone
3 Precentral gyrus
4 Superior frontal gyrus
5 Central sulcus
6 Caudate nucleus
7 Internal capsule
8 Lentiform nucleus
9 Thalamus
10 Orbital gyri
11 Lateral ventricle (choroid plexus)
12 Frontal sinus
13 Parietooccipital sulcus
14 Optic tract
15 Cerebral peduncle
16 Middle cerebral artery
17 Posterior cerebral artery
18 Occipital gyri
19 Uncus of hippocampal gyrus
20 Ethmoid labyrinth
21 Tentorium of cerebellum
22 Sphenoid sinus
23 Occipital bone

24 Internal carotid artery
25 Transverse sinus
26 Dentate nucleus
27 Clivus
28 Hard palate
29 Cerebellar tonsil
30 Nasopharynx
31 Longus capitis muscle
32 Rectus capitis posterior muscle (major)
33 Semispinalis capitis muscle
34 Oropharynx
35 Splenius capitis muscle
36 Genioglossus muscle
37 Sublingual gland
38 Trapezius muscle
39 Mandible (body)
40 Obliquus capitis inferior muscle
41 Geniohyoid muscle
42 Vertebral artery
43 Semispinalis cervicis muscle
44 Mylohyoid muscle
45 Hyoid bone

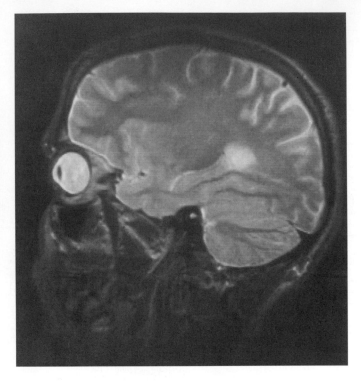

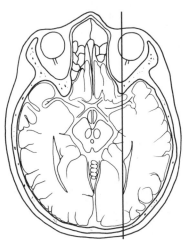

Frontal lobe

Temporal lobe

Parietal lobe

Occipital lobe

Cerebellum

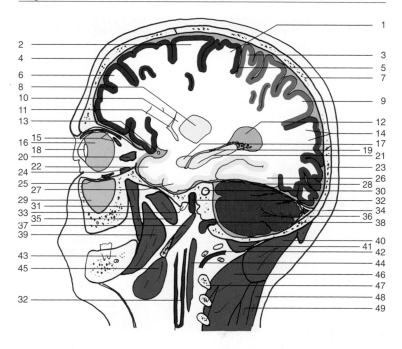

1 Precentral gyrus
2 Superior frontal gyrus
3 Postcentral gyrus
4 Frontal bone
5 Central sulcus
6 Frontal gyri
7 Parietal bone
8 Globus pallidus
9 Angular gyrus
10 Internal capsule
11 Putamen
12 Lateral ventricle
13 Middle cerebral artery
14 Occipital gyri
15 Superior rectus and
    levator palpebrae superioris muscles
16 Ocular bulb
17 Amygdaloid body
18 Lens
19 Lateral ventricle (temporal horn)
20 Lateral rectus muscle
21 Hippocampus
22 Middle temporal gyrus
23 Occipital bone
24 Orbital muscle

25 Inferior rectus muscle
26 Medial occipitotemporal gyrus
27 Inferior temporal gyrus
28 Tentorium of cerebellum
29 Maxillary sinus
30 Internal auditory canal
31 Temporal muscle
32 Internal carotid artery
33 Auditory tube (eustachian)
34 Transverse sinus
35 Lateral pterygoid muscle
36 Cerebellum (hemisphere)
37 Stylohyoid muscle
38 Internal jugular vein
39 Medial pterygoid muscle
40 Splenius capitis muscle
41 Rectus capitis muscle
42 Vertebral artery
43 Mandible
44 Longus colli muscle
45 Digastricus muscle (posterior belly)
46 Multifidus muscles
47 Transverse process
48 Trapezius muscle
49 Levator scapulae muscle

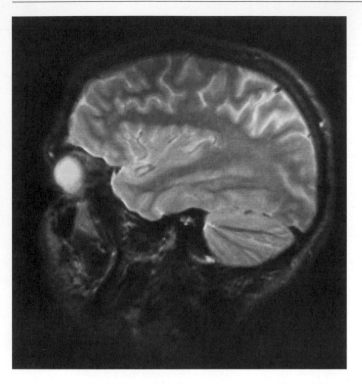

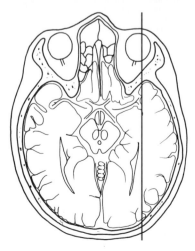

	Frontallappen	Frontal lobe
	Temporallappen	Temporal lobe
	Parietallappen	Parietal lobe
	Okzipitallappen	Occipital lobe
	Zerebellum	Cerebellum

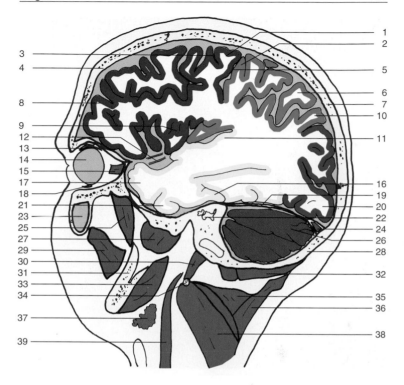

1 Precentral gyrus
2 Postcentral gyrus
3 Precentral sulcus
4 Frontal bone
5 Central sulcus
6 Supramarginal gyrus
7 Parietal bone
8 Inferior frontal gyrus
9 Insular lobe (cortex)
10 Angular gyrus
11 Transverse temporal gyri (Heschl's
   convolutions)
12 Lateral sulcus and insular arteries
13 Levator palpebrae superioris muscle
14 Ocular bulb
15 Lateral rectus muscle
16 Lateral occipitotemporal gyrus
17 Middle temporal gyrus
18 Inferior oblique muscle
19 Tentorium of cerebellum

20 Occipital gyri
21 Inferior temporal gyrus
22 Cochlea
23 Maxillary sinus
24 Transverse sinus
25 Temporal muscle
26 Cerebellum (caudal lobe)
27 Lateral pterygoid muscle
28 Occipital bone
29 Masseter muscle
30 Rectus capitis lateralis muscle
31 Mandible
32 Obliquus capitis muscle
33 Medial pterygoid muscle
34 Atlas (transverse process)
35 Longissimus capitis muscle
36 Splenius capitis muscle
37 Submandibular gland
38 Levator scapulae muscle
39 Jugular vein

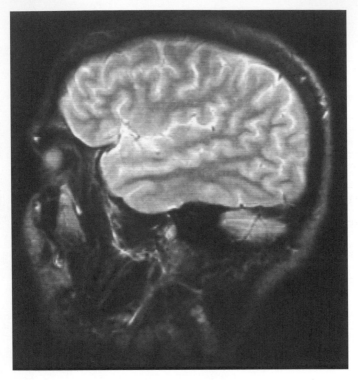

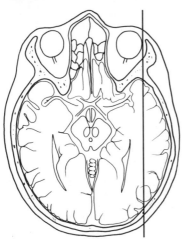

■ Frontal lobe
□ Temporal lobe
■ Parietal lobe
■ Cerebellum

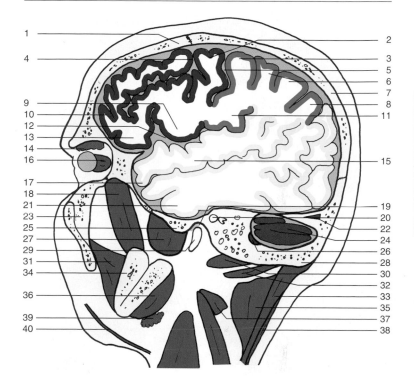

1 Frontal bone
2 Precentral gyrus
3 Postcentral gyrus
4 Precentral sulcus
5 Central sulcus
6 Supramarginal gyrus
7 Parietal bone
8 Angular gyrus
9 Frontal operculum
10 Inferior frontal gyrus
11 Parietal operculum
12 Lateral sulcus
13 Orbital gyri
14 Lacrimal gland
15 Superior temporal gyrus
16 Lateral rectus muscle
17 Middle temporal gyrus
18 Temporal muscle
19 Articular disk in mandibular fossa
20 Cochlea

21 Inferior temporal gyrus
22 Transverse sinus
23 Zygomatic bone
24 Cerebellum (caudal lobe)
25 Articular tubercle
26 Sigmoid sinus
27 Lateral pterygoid muscle
28 Occipital bone
29 Condyle of mandible
30 Rectus capitis lateralis muscle
31 Masseter muscle
32 Digastric muscle
33 Splenius capitis muscle
34 Mandible
35 Longissimus capitis muscle
36 Medial pterygoid muscle
37 Levator scapulae muscle
38 Trapezius muscle
39 Submandibular gland
40 Platysma

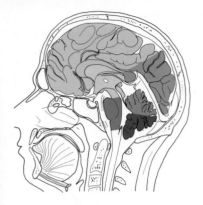
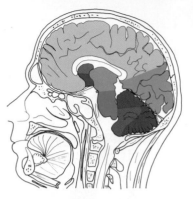
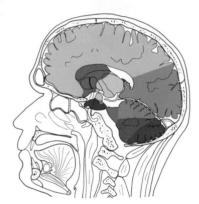
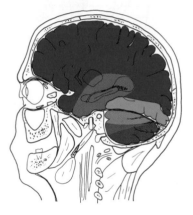

Anterior cerebral artery
- Terminal branches
- Central branches

Middle cerebral artery
- Terminal branches
- Central branches

Posterior cerebral artery
- Terminal branches
- Central branches
- Superior cerebellar artery
- Posterior inferior cerebellar artery
- Anterior inferior cerebellar artery
- Paramedian and circumferential arteries

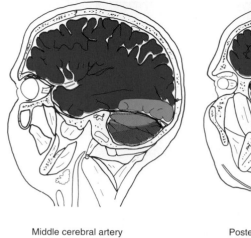

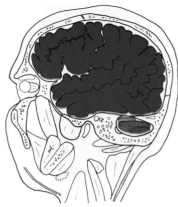

Middle cerebral artery
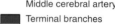 Terminal branches

Posterior cerebral artery
▨ Terminal branches
▨ Superior cerebellar artery
▨ Posterior inferior cerebellar artery
▨ Anterior inferior cerebellar artery

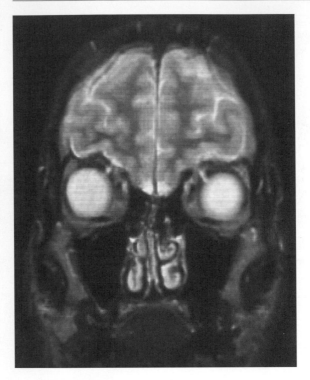

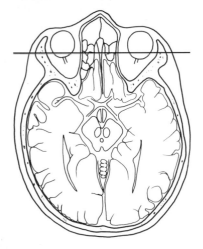

Frontal lobe

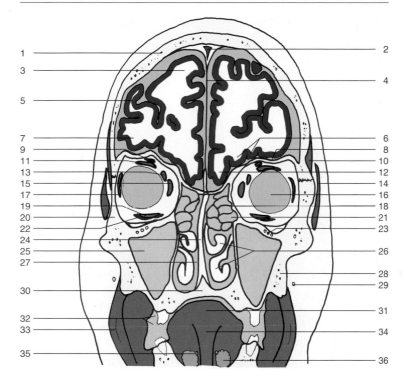

1 Frontal bone
2 Superior sagittal sinus
3 Superior frontal gyrus
4 Falx of cerebrum
5 Middle frontal gyrus
6 Orbital gyri
7 Inferior temporal gyrus
8 Orbital roof
9 Levator palpebrae superioris muscle
10 Temporal muscle
11 Superior rectus muscle
12 Straight gyrus
13 Superior oblique muscle
14 Orbicularis oculi muscle
15 Medial rectus muscle
16 Ocular bulb
17 Lateral rectus muscle
18 Lamina papyracea

19 Inferior rectus muscle
20 Zygomatic bone
21 Ethmoid labyrinth
22 Inferior oblique muscle
23 Infraorbital artery, vein, and nerve
24 Nasal septum
25 Maxillary sinus
26 Nasal conchae, middle and inferior
27 Nasal cavity
28 Maxilla
29 Parotid duct
30 Hard palate
31 Tongue
32 Oral cavity
33 Depressor anguli oris muscle
34 Genioglossus muscle
35 Submandibular duct
36 Sublingual gland

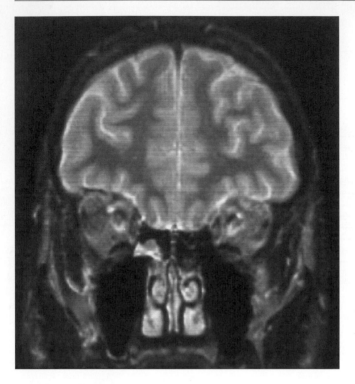

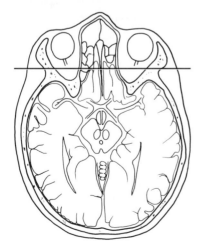

Frontal lobe

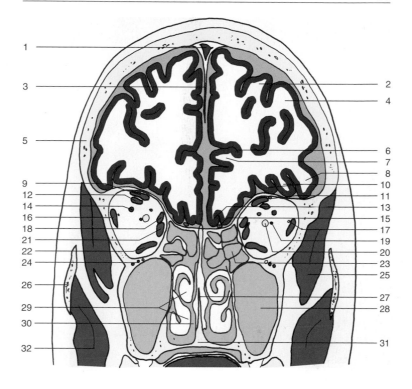

1 Superior sagittal sinus
2 Superior frontal gyrus
3 Falx of cerebrum
4 Middle frontal gyrus
5 Frontal bone
6 Cingulate sulcus
7 Cingulate gyrus
8 Inferior frontal gyrus
9 Levator palpebrae superioris muscle
10 Orbital gyri
11 Trochlear nerve
12 Superior rectus muscle
13 Straight gyrus
14 Superior ophtalmic vein
15 Olfactoric tract
16 Lateral rectus muscle

17 Abducens nerve
18 Superior oblique muscle
19 Ophthalmic artery
20 Optic nerve
21 Medial rectus muscle
22 Inferior rectus muscle
23 Ethmoid labyrinth
24 Infraorbital nerve, artery and vein
25 Temporal muscle
26 Zygomatic arch
27 Nasal septum
28 Maxillary sinus
29 Nasal conchae
30 Nasal cavity
31 Hard palate
32 Masseter muscle

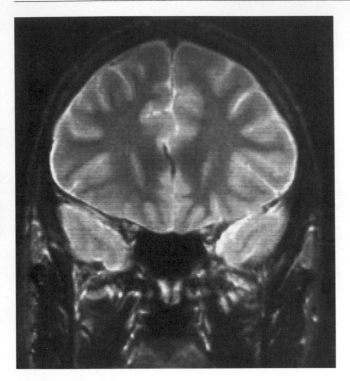

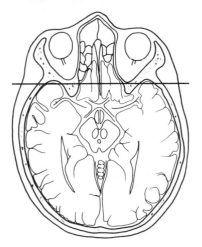

■ Frontal lobe
□ Temporal lobe

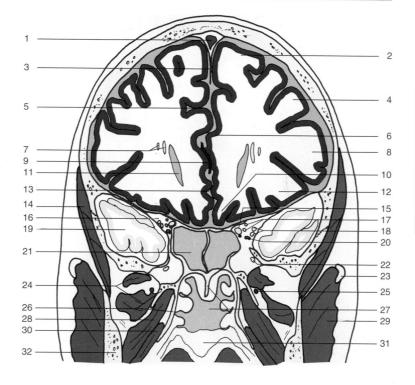

1 Superior sagittal sinus
2 Superior frontal gyrus
3 Falx of cerebrum
4 Middle frontal gyrus
5 Cingulate sulcus
6 Cingulate gyrus
7 Lentiform nucleus
8 Inferior frontal gyrus
9 Anterior cerebral artery
10 Straight gyrus
11 Lateral ventricle (frontal horn)
12 Orbital gyrus
13 Anterior longitudinal fissure
14 Temporal muscle
15 Optic nerve (CN II)
16 Superior orbital fissure
17 Trochlear and oculomotor nerves
18 Ophthalmic (first trigeminal branch) and abducens nerves
19 Temporal lobe (anterior pole)
20 Ophthalmic artery and vein
21 Sphenoid sinus
22 Maxillary nerve
23 Zygomatic arch
24 Lateral pterygoid muscle
25 Maxillary artery
26 Pterygoid process (lateral and medial plates)
27 Nasal septum and cavity
28 Medial pterygoid muscle
29 Masseter muscle
30 Tensor veli palatini muscle
31 Soft palate
32 Mandible (ramus)

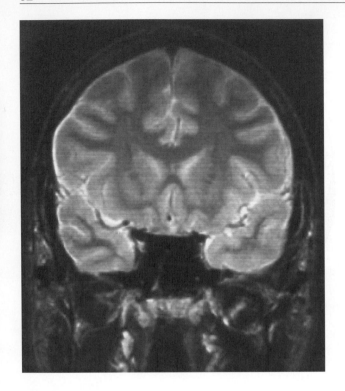

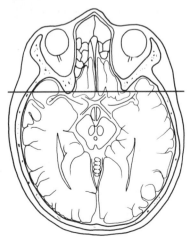

■ Frontal lobe
□ Temporal lobe

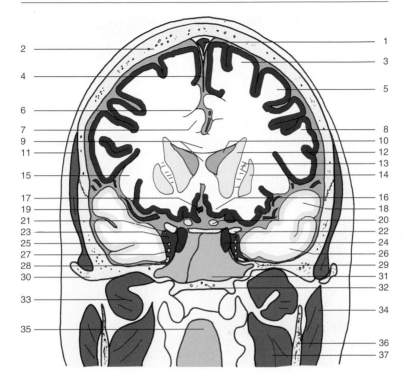

1 Superior sagittal sinus
2 Parietal bone
3 Superior frontal gyrus
4 Falx of cerebrum
5 Middle frontal gyrus
6 Cingulate sulcus
7 Cingulate gyrus
8 Inferior frontal gyrus
9 Corpus callosum (genu)
10 Lateral ventricle (anterior horn)
11 Temporal muscle
12 Caudate nucleus (head)
13 Internal capsule
14 Putamen
15 Insular lobe
16 Straight gyrus
17 Anterior cerebral artery
18 Superior temporal gyrus
19 Insular arteries
20 Optic nerve (CN II)

21 Oculomotor nerve (CN III)
22 Anterior clinoid process
23 Trochlear nerve (CN IV)
24 Internal carotid artery
25 Ophthalmic nerve (first trigeminal branch)
26 Middle temporal gyrus
27 Abducens nerve (CN VI)
28 Maxillary nerve (second trigeminal branch)
29 Cavernous sinus
30 Zygomatic arch
31 Sphenoid sinus
32 Sphenoid bone
33 Lateral pterygoid muscle
34 Masseter muscle
35 Nasopharynx
36 Mandible (ramus)
37 Medial pterygoid muscle

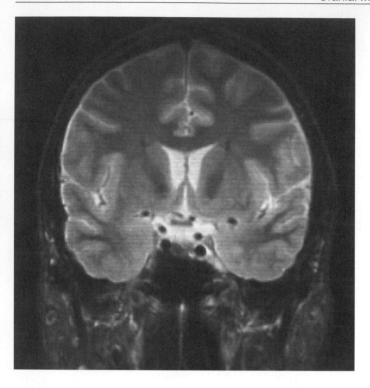

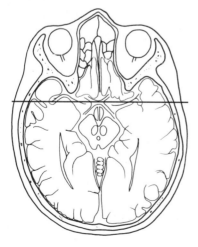

■ Frontal lobe
□ Temporal lobe

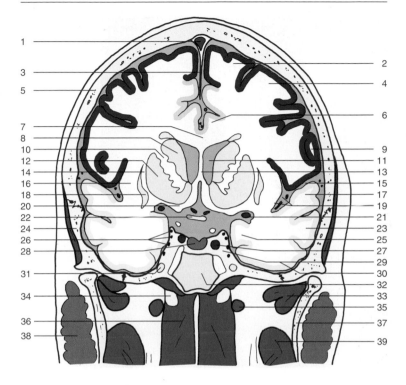

1 Superior sagittal sinus
2 Superior frontal gyrus
3 Falx of cerebrum
4 Middle frontal gyrus
5 Parietal bone
6 Cingulate sulcus
7 Corpus callosum (body)
8 Caudate nucleus (head)
9 Inferior frontal gyrus
10 Internal capsule (anterior crus)
11 Lateral ventricle (anterior horn)
12 Putamen
13 Pellucid septum
14 External capsule
15 Lateral sulcus
16 Extreme capsule
17 Superior temporal gyrus
18 Claustrum
19 Insular lobe and insular cistern
20 Roof of chiasmatic cistern

21 Middle cerebral artery
22 Optic chiasm
23 Middle temporal gyrus
24 Temporal bone
25 Parahippocampal gyrus
26 Oculomotor (CN II), trochlear (CN IV), and abducens (CN VI) nerves
27 Internal carotid artery
28 Pituitary gland
29 Cavernous sinus
30 Lateral occipitotemporal gyrus
31 Trigeminal ganglion
32 Sphenoid sinus
33 Lateral pterygoid muscle
34 Auditory tube
35 Levator veli palatini muscle
36 Nasopharynx (constrictor muscle)
37 Mandible (ramus)
38 Parotid gland
39 Medial pterygoid muscle

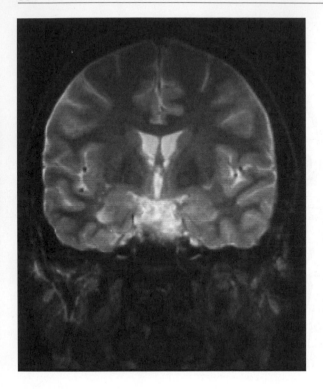

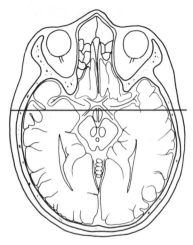

■ Frontal lobe
☐ Temporal lobe

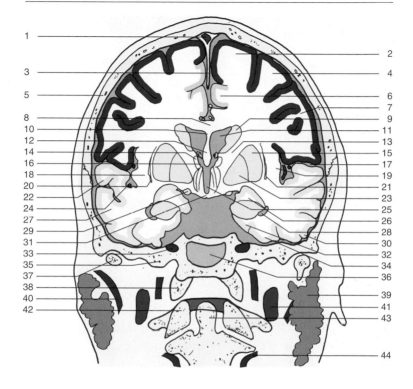

1 Superior sagittal sinus
2 Superior frontal gyrus
3 Falx of cerebrum
4 Middle frontal gyrus
5 Parietal bone
6 Cingulate gyrus
7 Precentral gyrus
8 Corpus callosum (body)
9 Caudate nucleus (body)
10 Pellucid septum
11 Lateral ventricle
12 Fornix
13 Internal capsule
14 Anterior thalamic nuclei
15 Putamen
16 Interventricular foramen (Monro's)
17 Lateral sulcus
18 Extreme capsule
19 Insular lobe
20 External capsule
21 Claustrum
22 Superior temporal gyrus

23 Globus pallidus
24 Insular cistern
25 Third ventricle
26 Amygdaloid body
27 Middle temporal gyrus
28 Lateral ventricle (temporal horn)
29 Optic tract
30 Inferior temporal gyrus
31 Mammillary body
32 Parahippocampal gyrus
33 Internal carotid artery
34 Lateral occipitotemporal gyrus
35 Sphenoid bone
36 Sphenoid sinus
37 Condyle of mandible
38 Occipital condyle
39 Parotid gland
40 External carotid artery
41 Internal jugular vein
42 Atlas (lateral mass)
43 Odontoid process of axis
44 Vertebral artery

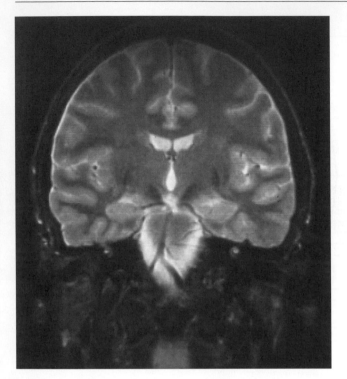

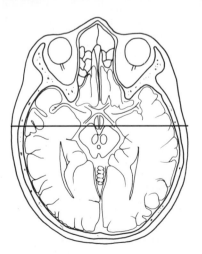

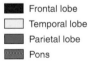

Frontal lobe
Temporal lobe
Parietal lobe
Pons

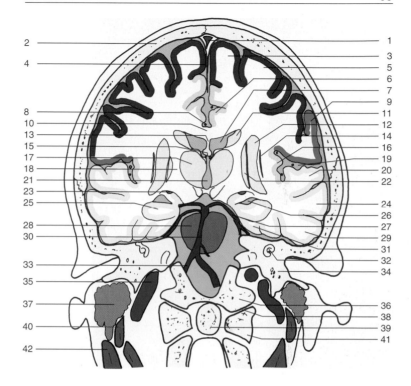

1 Superior sagittal sinus
2 Parietal bone
3 Superior frontal gyrus
4 Falx of cerebrum
5 Middle frontal gyrus
6 Cingulate gyrus
7 Lateral ventricle
8 Pericallosal artery
9 Precentral gyrus
10 Corpus callosum (body)
11 Caudate nucleus (head)
12 Putamen
13 Pellucid septum
14 Claustrum
15 Fornix
16 Insular lobe
17 Thalamus
18 Internal capsule
19 Lateral sulcus
20 Superior temporal gyrus
21 Third ventricle

22 Globus pallidus
23 Optic tract
24 Middle temporal gyrus
25 Hippocampus
26 Lateral ventricle (temporal horn)
27 Posterior cerebral artery
28 Pons
29 Inferior temporal gyrus
30 Basilar artery
31 Parahippocampal gyrus
32 Cochlea
33 Vertebral artery
34 Temporal bone
35 Internal jugular vein
36 Occipital condyle
37 Parotid gland
38 Atlantooccipital articulation
39 Odontoid process of axis
40 Digastric muscle (posterior belly)
41 Atlas (lateral mass)
42 Sternocleidomastoid muscle

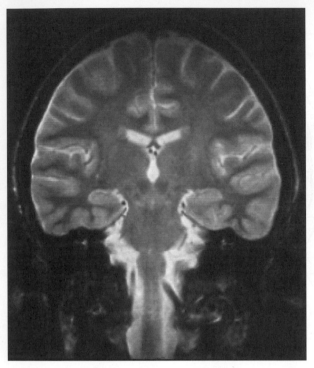

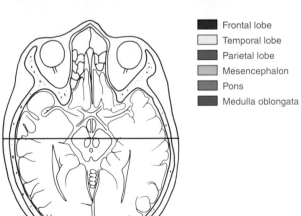

■ Frontal lobe
□ Temporal lobe
■ Parietal lobe
■ Mesencephalon
■ Pons
■ Medulla oblongata

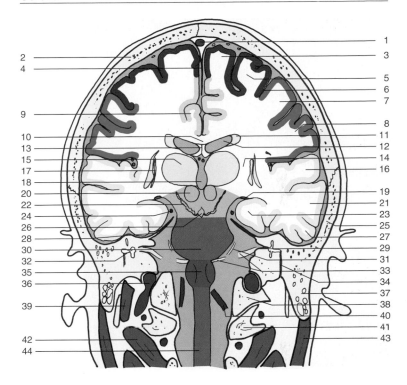

1 Superior sagittal sinus
2 Parietal bone
3 Superior frontal gyrus
4 Falx of cerebrum
5 Precentral gyrus
6 Central sulcus
7 Postcentral gyrus
8 Supramarginal gyrus
9 Cingulate gyrus
10 Corpus callosum (body)
11 Caudate nucleus
12 Lateral ventricle
13 Fornix
14 Internal capsule
15 Thalamus
16 Superior temporal gyrus
17 Lentiform nucleus
    (putamen, globus pallidus)
18 Third ventricle
19 Optic tract
20 Red nucleus
21 Middle temporal gyrus
22 Black substance

23 Parahippocampal gyrus
24 Posterior cerebral artery
25 Temporal bone
26 Interpeduncular cistern
27 Inferior temporal gyrus
28 Tentorium of cerebellum
29 Internal auditory canal
30 Pons
31 Trigeminal nerve
32 Cochlea
33 Vestibulocochlear nerve
34 Facial canal
35 Medulla oblongata
36 Internal jugular vein
37 Mastoid process
38 Occipital condyle
39 Digastric muscle
40 Vertebral artery
41 Atlas (lateral mass)
42 Obliquus capitis muscle
43 Sternocleidomastoid muscle
44 Spinal cord

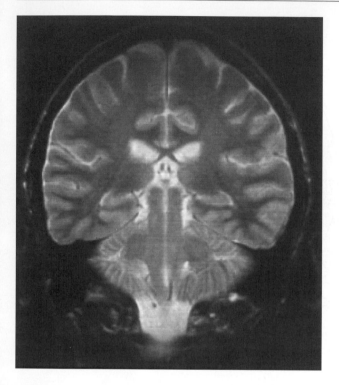

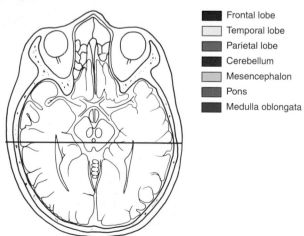

- ■ Frontal lobe
- □ Temporal lobe
- ■ Parietal lobe
- ■ Cerebellum
- ■ Mesencephalon
- ▨ Pons
- ■ Medulla oblongata

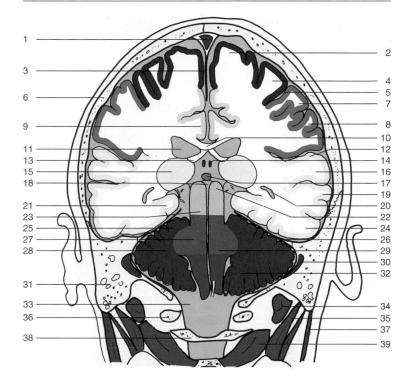

1 Superior sagittal sinus
2 Superior frontal gyrus
3 Falx of cerebrum
4 Precentral gyrus
5 Central sulcus
6 Parietal bone
7 Postcentral gyrus
8 Supramarginal gyrus
9 Cingulate gyrus
10 Corpus callosum
11 Lateral ventricle
12 Transverse temporal gyri
(Heschl's convolutions)
13 Fornix
14 Internal cerebral vein
15 Thalamus
16 Superior temporal gyrus
17 Pineal body
18 Aqueduct (aperture)
19 Middle temporal gyrus

20 Lateral ventricle (temporal horn)
21 Parahippocampal gyrus
22 Cranial colliculus
23 Mesencephalon
24 Inferior temporal gyrus
25 Cerebellum (cranial lobe)
26 Tentorium of cerebellum
27 Roof of fourth ventricle
28 Middle cerebellar peduncle
29 Pons
30 Sigmoid sinus
31 Mastoid process
32 Floccule
33 Cerebellomedullary cistern
34 Obliquus capitis superior muscle
35 Rectus capitis superior muscle
36 Atlas (posterior arch)
37 Sternocleidomastoid muscle
38 Axis
39 Obliquus capitis inferior muscle

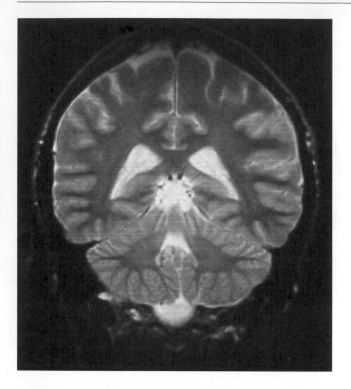

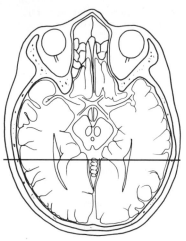

■ Frontal lobe
☐ Temporal lobe
■ Parietal lobe
■ Cerebellum

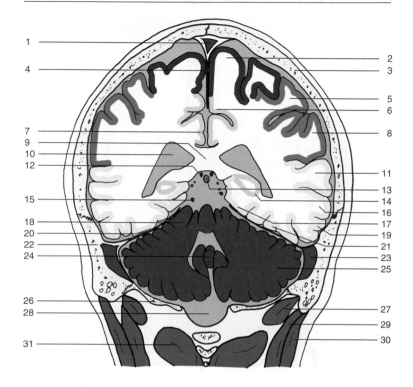

1 Superior sagittal sinus
2 Superior frontal gyrus
3 Parietal bone
4 Falx of cerebrum
5 Postcentral gyrus
6 Paracentral lobule
7 Cingulate gyrus
8 Supramarginal gyrus
9 Corpus callosum (splenium)
10 Lateral ventricle (posterior horn)
11 Superior temporal gyrus
12 Internal cerebral vein
13 Pineal body
14 Hippocampus
15 Superior cerebellar artery
16 Middle temporal gyrus
17 Medial occipitotemporal gyrus
18 Cerebellum (cranial lobe)
19 Inferior temporal gyrus
20 Tentorium of cerebellum
21 Lateral occipitotemporal gyrus
22 Temporal bone
23 Sigmoid sinus
24 Uvula vermis
25 Cerebellum (caudal lobe)
26 Occipital bone
27 Obliquus capitis superior muscle
28 Cerebellomedullary cistern
29 Longissimus capitis muscle
30 Splenius capitis muscle
31 Obliquus capitis inferior muscle

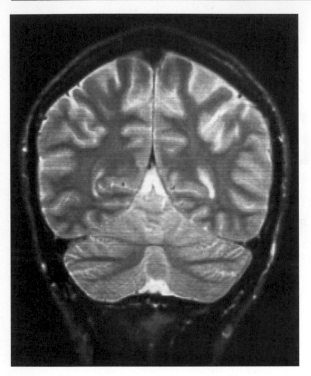

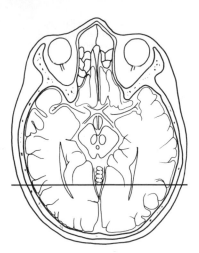

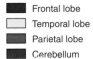

Frontal lobe
Temporal lobe
Parietal lobe
Cerebellum

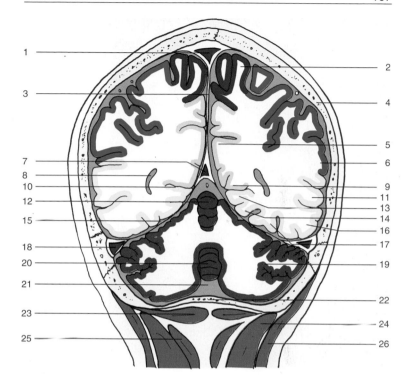

1 Superior sagittal sinus
2 Superior parietal lobule
3 Falx of cerebrum
4 Parietal bone
5 Precuneus
6 Angular gyrus
7 Straight sinus
8 Lateral ventricle (posterior horn)
9 Cuneus
10 Calcarine sulcus
11 Middle temporal gyrus
12 Cerebellum (cranial lobe)
13 Striate cortex

14 Medial occipitotemporal gyrus
15 Tentorium of cerebellum
16 Inferior temporal gyrus
17 Lateral temporal gyrus
18 Transverse sinus
19 Cerebellum (caudal lobe)
20 Pyramis vermis
21 Cerebellomedullary cistern
22 Occipital bone
23 Rectus capitis posterior muscle (minor)
24 Semispinalis capitis muscle
25 Rectus capitis posterior muscle (major)
26 Splenius capitis muscle

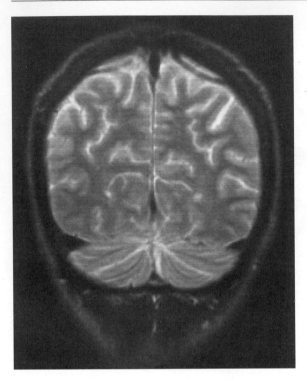

Parietal lobe
Occipital lobe
Cerebellum

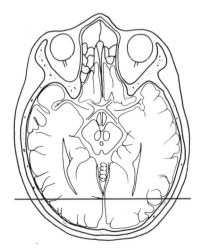

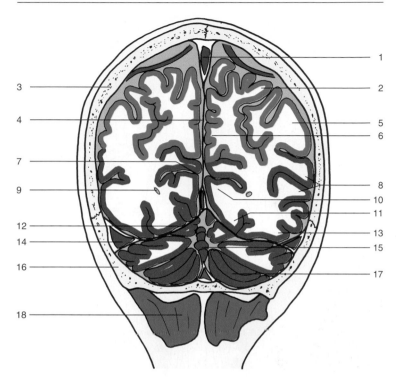

1 Superior sagittal sinus
2 Superior parietal lobule
3 Parietal bone
4 Falx of cerebrum
5 Angular gyrus
6 Precuneus
7 Calcarine sulcus
8 Occipital gyri
9 Lateral ventricle (posterior horn)
10 Cuneus
11 Medial occipitotemporal gyrus
12 Tentorium of cerebellum
13 Lateral occipitotemporal gyrus
14 Transverse sinus
15 Vermis of cerebellum
16 Occipital bone
17 Cerebellum (caudal lobe)
18 Semispinalis capitis muscle

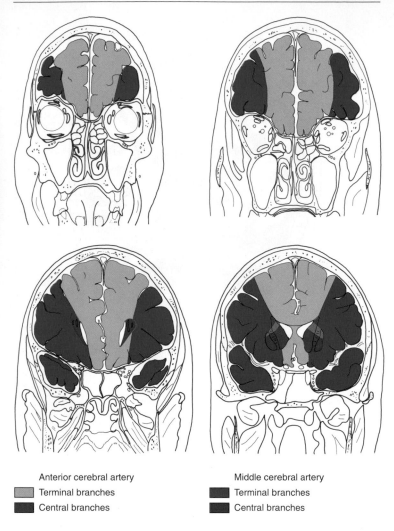

Anterior cerebral artery
- Terminal branches
- Central branches

Middle cerebral artery
- Terminal branches
- Central branches

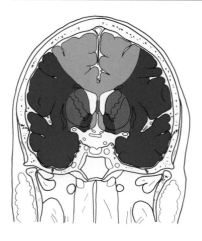

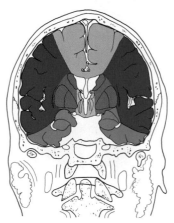

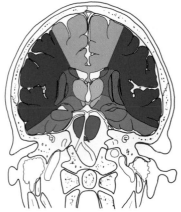

Anterior cerebral artery
- Terminal branches
- Central branches

Middle cerebral artery
- Terminal branches
- Central branches

Posterior cerebral artery
- Terminal branches
- Central branches
- Paramedian and circumferential arteries

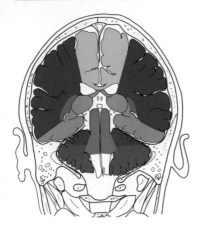

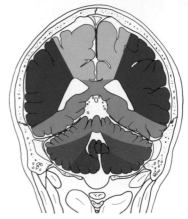

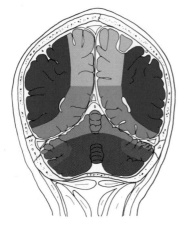

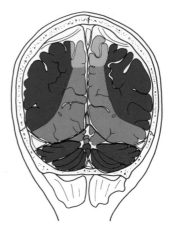

Anterior cerebral artery
- Terminal branches
- Central branches

Middle cerebral artery
- Terminal branches
- Central branches

Posterior cerebral artery
- Terminal branches
- Centrale branches
- Superior cerebellar artery
- Posterior inferior cerebellar artery
- Anterior inferior cerebellar artery
- Paramedian and circumferential arteries

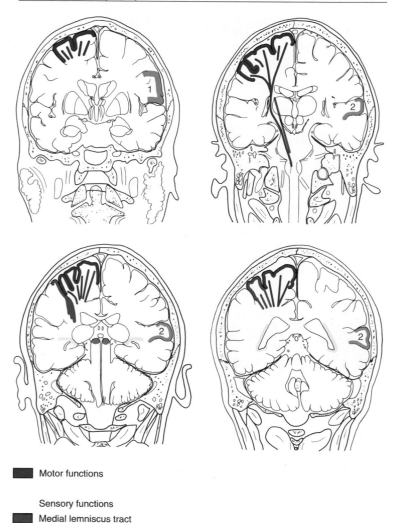

Motor functions

Sensory functions
Medial lemniscus tract
Spinothalamic tract
Mesencephalic nucleus of trigeminal nerve

Oculomotor nucleus and tract
Optic tract
Speech area (1=motor, 2=sensory)

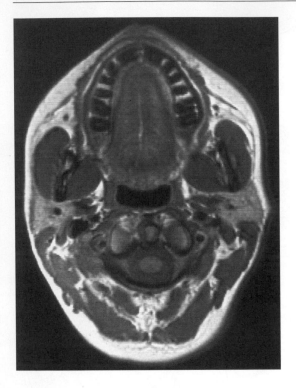

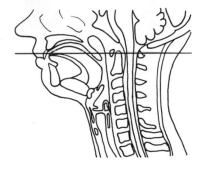

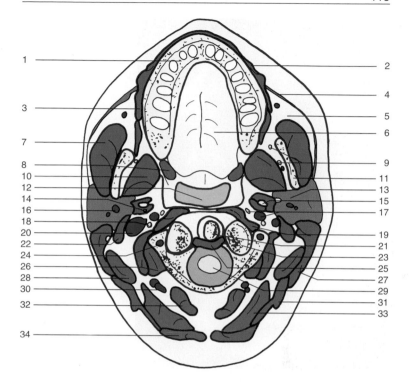

1 Maxillary bone (alveolar process)
2 Orbicularis oris muscle
3 Depressor anguli oris muscle
4 Parotid duct
5 Retromolar fossa
6 Hard palate
7 Masseter muscle
8 Palatine tonsil, superior constrictor muscle of pharynx
9 Inferior alveolar nerve, lingual nerve
10 Medial pterygoid muscle
11 Mandible
12 Nasopharynx
13 Parotid gland
14 Accessory nerve (CN XI)
15 Styloid process and styloid muscles
16 Retromandibular vein
17 Internal carotid artery and hypoglossal nerve (CN XII)

18 Glossopharyngeal (CN IX) and vagus (CN X) nerves
19 Longus capitis muscle
20 Internal jugular vein
21 Odontoid process of axis
22 Digastric muscle (posterior belly)
23 Atlas (lateral mass)
24 Vertebral artery
25 Cruciform ligament of atlas
26 Obliquus capitis inferior and superior muscles
27 Sternocleidomastoid muscle
28 Longus capitis muscle
29 Spinal cord
30 Deep cervical vein
31 Splenius capitis muscle
32 Rectus capitis posterior muscle (major)
33 Semispinalis capitis muscle
34 Trapezius muscle

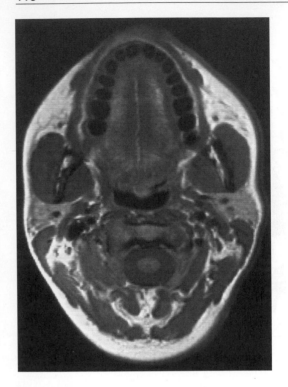

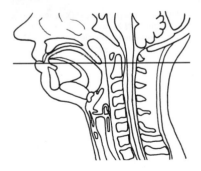

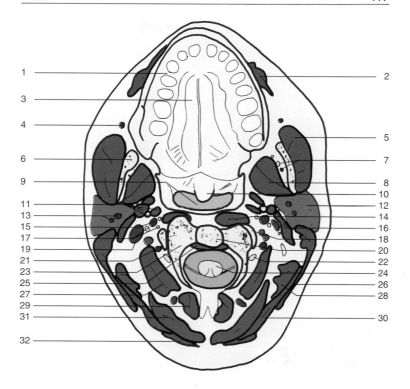

1 Maxillary bone (alveolar process)
2 Zygomaticus major muscle
3 Hard palate
4 Facial artery
5 Masseter muscle
6 Mandible (ramus)
7 Lingual and inferior alveolar nerves
8 Medial pterygoid muscle
9 Nasopharynx
10 Uvula and soft palate
11 Styloid process and styloid muscles
12 Parotid gland
13 Superficial temporal artery and retromandibular vein
14 Longus capitis muscle
15 Internal carotid artery
16 Digastric muscle (posterior belly)
17 Vagus (CN X) and hypoglossal (CN XII) nerves
18 Atlas (anterior arch)
19 Internal jugular vein
20 Odontoid process of axis
21 Vertebral artery
22 Posterior root of spinal nerve C2
23 Axis (body)
24 Spinal cord
25 Transverse ligament of atlas
26 Sternocleidomastoid muscle
27 Obliquus capitis inferior muscle
28 Longissimus capitis muscle
29 Rectus capitis posterior muscle (major)
30 Splenius capitis muscle
31 Semispinalis capitis muscle
32 Trapezius muscle

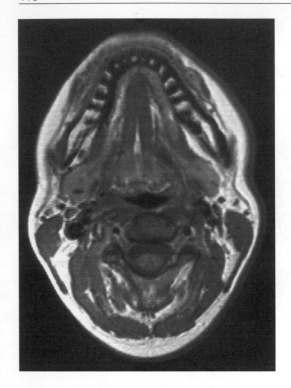

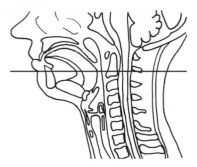

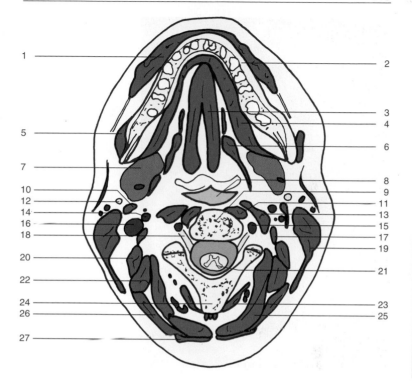

1 Depressor anguli oris muscle
2 Mandible (body)
3 Genioglossus muscle
4 Mylohyoid muscle
5 Masseter muscle
6 Hyoglossus muscle
7 Submandibular gland
8 Oropharynx
9 Axis (body)
10 Digastric muscle (posterior belly)
11 Longus colli muscle
12 Auriculotemporal nerve (branch)
13 Longus capitis muscle
14 Internal carotid artery

15 Vertebral artery
16 Internal jugular vein
17 Splenius cervicis muscle
18 Root of nerve C3
19 Sternocleidomastoid muscle
20 Levator scapulae muscle
21 Spinal cord
22 Longissimus cervicis muscle
23 Obliquus capitis inferior muscle
24 Spinous process
25 Semispinalis capitis muscle
26 Splenius capitis muscle
27 Trapezius muscle

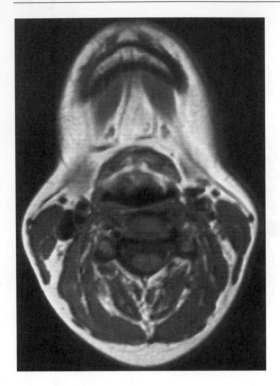

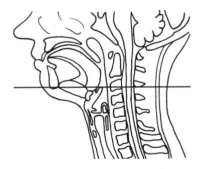

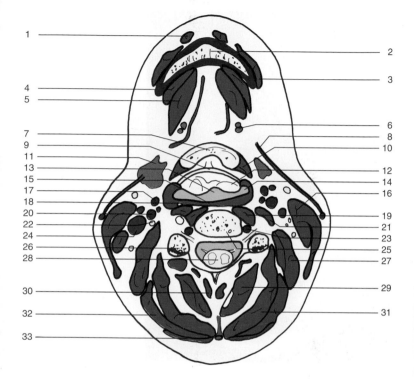

1 Mentalis muscle
2 Mandible
3 Depressor anguli oris muscle
4 Mylohyoid muscle
5 Geniohyoid muscle
6 Sublingual gland
7 Hyoid bone
8 Platysma
9 Epiglottis
10 Infrahyoid (strap) muscles
11 Submandibular gland
12 Aryepiglottic fold
13 Larynx
14 Piriform sinus
15 Inferior constrictor muscle of pharynx
   and retropharyngeal space
16 Sternocleidomastoid muscle
17 External carotid artery

18 Sympathetic trunk
19 Longus colli muscle
20 Internal carotid artery
21 Anterior scalene muscle
22 Vagus nerve
23 Vertebral artery
24 Internal jugular vein
25 Cervical vertebra 4
26 Articular facet C3/4
27 Levator scapulae and
   longissimus capitis muscles
28 Spinal cord
29 Semispinalis cervicis muscle
30 Multifidus muscles
31 Semispinalis capitis muscle
32 Splenius capitis muscle
33 Trapezius muscle

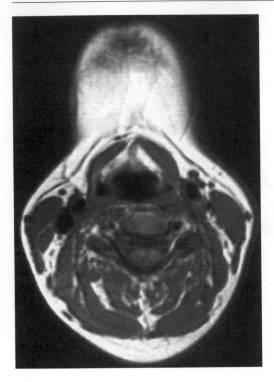

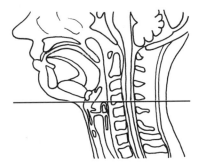

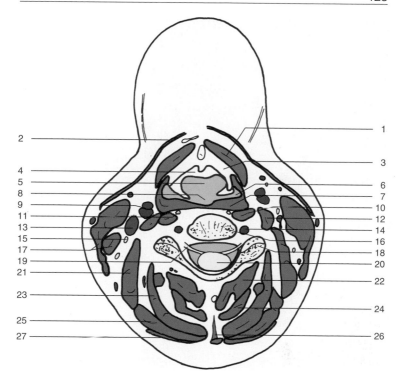

1 Infrahyoid (strap) muscles
(sternohyoid and sternothyroid muscles)
2 Platysma
3 Thyroid cartilage
4 Epiglottis
5 Larynx
6 Piriform sinus
7 Inferior constrictor muscle of pharynx
8 Hypopharynx
9 Carotid artery (bifurcation)
10 Longus colli muscle
11 Sympathetic trunk
12 Anterior scalene muscle
13 Internal jugular vein

14 Vertebral artery
15 Vagus nerve
16 Cervical vertebra 4
17 Sternocleidomastoid muscle
18 Articular facet C4/5
19 Spinalis muscle
20 Spinal cord
21 Levator scapulae muscle
22 Multifidus muscles
23 Semispinalis capitis muscle
24 Semispinalis cervicis muscle
25 Splenius capitis muscle
26 Nuchal ligament
27 Trapezius muscle

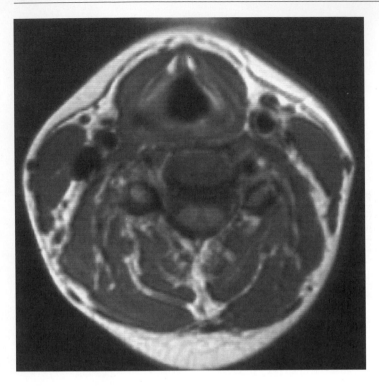

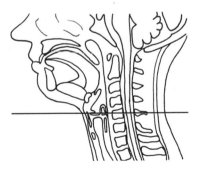

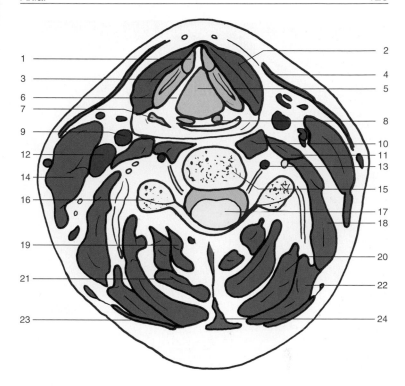

1 Thyroid cartilage (lamina)
2 Infrahyoid (strap) muscles (sternohyoid, thyrohyoid, sternothyroid, omohyoid muscles)
3 Thyroid cartilage
4 Platysma
5 Larynx (vestibule)
6 Vestibular fold
7 Piriform sinus
8 Arytenoid cartilage
9 Common carotid artery
10 Anterior scalene muscle
11 Longus colli muscle
12 Jugular vein
13 Vertebral artery
14 Sternocleidomastoid muscle
15 Cervical vertebra 5
16 Articular facet C5/6
17 Spinal cord
18 Levator scapulae muscle
19 Multifidus muscles
20 Semispinalis capitis muscle
21 Semispinalis cervicis muscle
22 Splenius capitis muscle
23 Trapezius muscle
24 Nuchal ligament

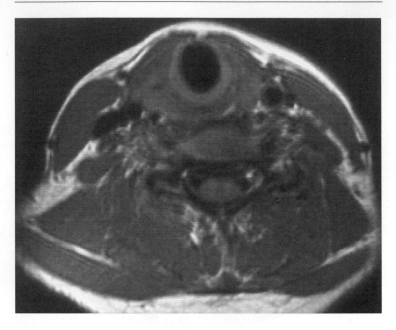

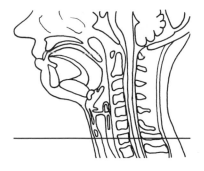

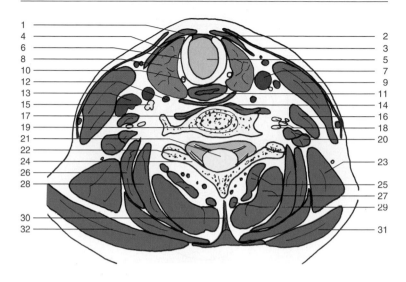

1 Sternohyoid muscle
2 Cricothyroid ligament
3 Platysma
4 Sternothyroid muscle
5 Infraglottic space
6 Cricoid cartilage
7 Common carotid artery
8 Thyroid gland
9 Sternocleidomastoid muscle
10 Thyroid cartilage, inferior horn
11 Pharynx (laryngeal part)
12 Vertebral artery
13 Internal jugular vein
14 Inferior constrictor muscle of pharynx
15 Vagus nerve (CN XI)
16 Anterior scalene muscle
17 Longus colli muscle

18 Brachial plexus
19 Cervical vertebra 7
20 Medial and posterior scalene muscles
21 Cervical spinal cord
22 Articular facet
23 Levator scapulae muscle
24 Arch of cervical vertebra 7
25 Multifidus muscles
26 Cervical iliocostalis muscle
27 Semispinalis cervicis muscle
28 Longissimus cervicis muscle
29 Spinalis muscle
30 Nuchal ligament
31 Splenius cervicis and splenius capitis muscles
32 Trapezius muscle

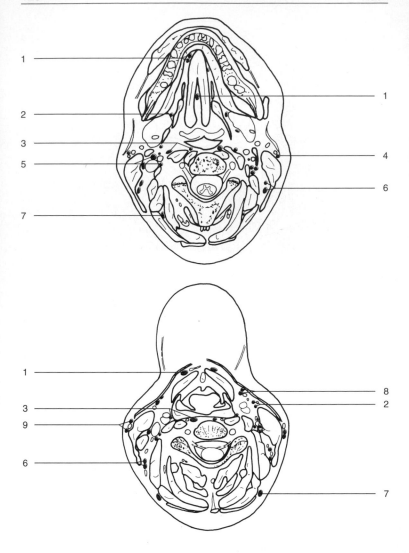

1 Submental lymph nodes
2 Submandibular lymph nodes
3 Retropharyngeal lymph nodes
4 Preauricular lymph nodes
5 Anterior and lateral jugular lymph nodes

6 Deep cervical lymph nodes
7 Nuchal lymph nodes
8 Anterior jugular lymph nodes
9 Superficial cervical lymph nodes

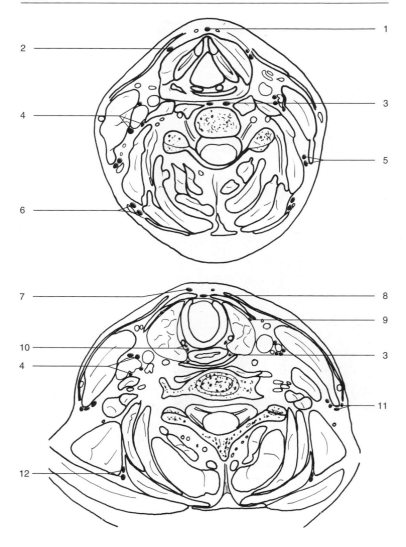

1 Prelaryngeal lymph nodes
2 Anterior jugular lymph nodes
3 Retropharyngeal lymph nodes
4 Inferior jugular group
5 Deep cervical lymph nodes
6 Nuchal lymph nodes

7 Anterior cervical lymph nodes
8 Pretracheal lymph nodes
9 Thyroid lymph nodes
10 Pretracheal lymph nodes
11 Supraclavicular lymph nodes
12 Superficial cervical lymph nodes

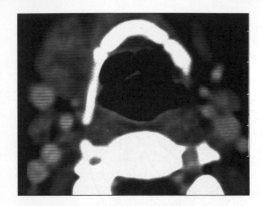

1

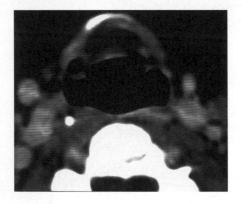

2

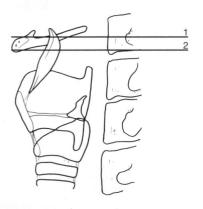

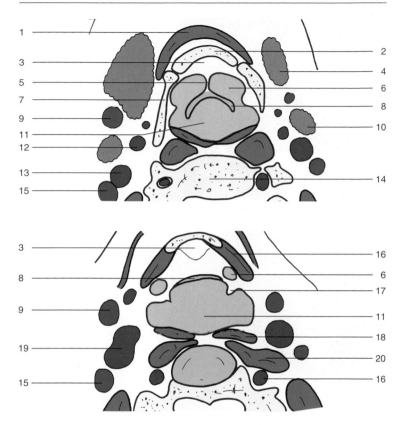

1 Infrahyoid (strap) muscles (mylohyoid, geniohyoid, and hyoglossus muscles)
2 Hyoid bone (body)
3 Preepiglottic space
4 Submandibular gland
5 Glossoepiglottic fold
6 Vallecula epiglottica
7 Hyoid bone (greater horn)
8 Epiglottis
9 Anterior jugular vein
10 Parotid gland
11 Hypopharynx
12 External carotid artery
13 Internal carotid artery
14 Cervical vertebra 3
15 Internal jugular vein
16 Infrahyoid muscles (sternohyoid and sternothyroid muscles)
17 Pharyngoepiglottic fold
18 Inferior constrictor muscle of pharynx
19 Carotid bifurcation
20 Longus colli muscle

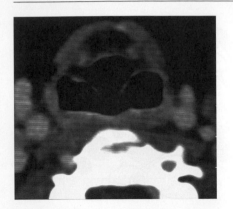

3

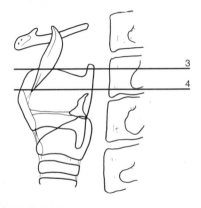

4

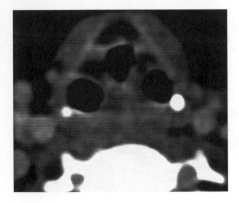

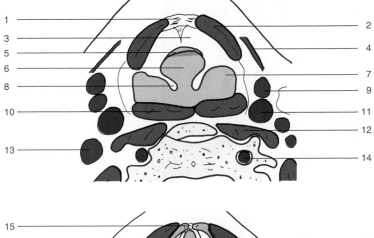

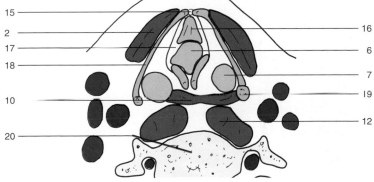

1 Thyrohyoid membrane
2 Infrahyoid (strap) muscles (sternothyroid, omohyoid, and thyrohyoid muscles)
3 Preepiglottic space
4 Platysma
5 Epiglottis
6 Larynx
7 Piriform sinus
8 Aryepiglottic fold
9 Anterior jugular vein
10 Inferior constrictor muscle of pharynx
11 Common carotid artery
12 Longus colli muscle
13 Internal jugular vein
14 Vertebral artery
15 Superior thyroid notch
16 Stem of epiglottis
17 Vestibular fold
18 Thyroid cartilage (lamina)
19 Thyroid cartilage (superior horn)
20 Cervical vertebra 4

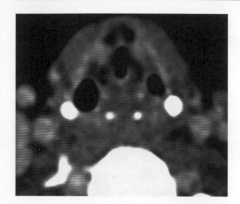

5

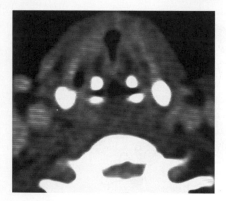

6

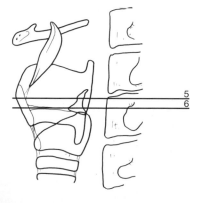

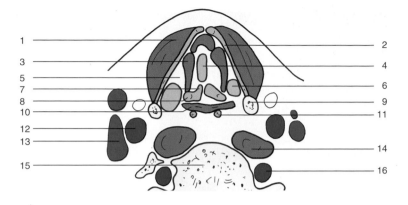

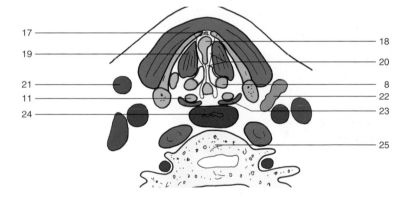

1 Infrahyoid (strap) muscles (sternothyroid, omohyoid, and thyrohyoid muscle)
2 Thyroid cartilage
3 Thyroarytenoid muscle
4 Larynx (vestibule)
5 Paralaryngeal space
6 Piriform sinus
7 Arytenoid cartilage (vocal process)
8 Arytenoid cartilage (body)
9 Thyroid cartilage (superior horn)
10 Transverse arytenoid muscle
11 Cricoid cartilage
12 Common carotid artery

13 Internal jugular vein
14 Longus colli muscle
15 Cervical vertebra 4
16 Vertebral artery
17 Laryngeal prominence
18 Fissure of glottis
19 Vocalis muscle
20 Vocal cord
21 Anterior jugular vein
22 Thyroid gland
23 Oblique arytenoid muscle
24 Esophagus
25 Cervical vertebra 5

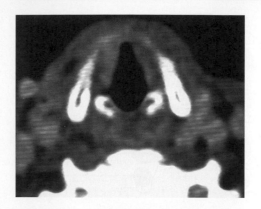

7

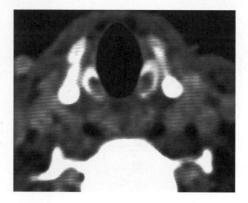

8

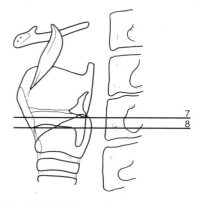

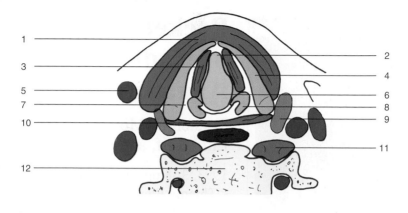

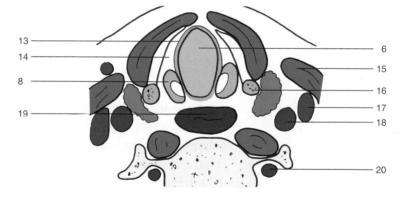

1 Infrahyoid (strap) muscles (sternohyoid
  and omohyoid muscles, sternothyroid
  muscle)
2 Anterior laryngeal commissure
3 Vocalis muscle
4 Thyroid cartilage
5 Anterior jugular vein
6 Subglottic space
7 Cricothyroid joint
8 Cricoid cartilage (lamina)
9 Thyroid gland

10 Inferior constrictor muscle of pharynx
11 Longus colli muscle
12 Cervical vertebra 5
13 Elastic cone
14 Paralaryngeal space
15 Sternocleidomastoid muscle
16 Thyroid cartilage (inferior horn)
17 Internal jugular vein
18 Common carotid artery
19 Esophagus
20 Vertebral artery

Pocket Atlas of Radiographic Anatomy

Torsten B. Möller,
Emil Reif, and Paul Stark

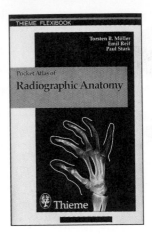

1993. 368 pp., 348 illustrations
<Thieme Flexibook>
ISBN 3 13 784201 8 (GTV, Stuttgart)
ISBN 0 86577 459 5 (TMP, New York)

This pocket atlas presents the anatomy seen in radiographs, including the many details that must be recognized in order to interpret the findings well. A radiograph example for each of 170 different projections in conventional radiography is shown and juxtaposed with a clearly labeled drawing that facilitates quick and sure finding of the anatomic structure being sought. In order to make this book useful in daily practice, radiologic "colloquialisms" are provided in addition to the regular anatomic terms.

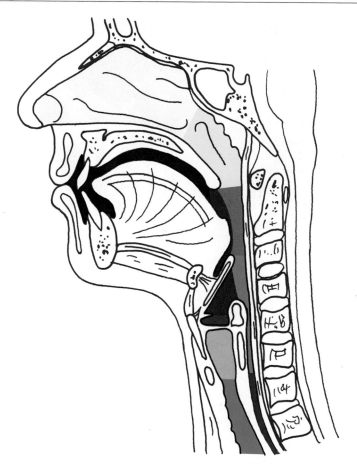

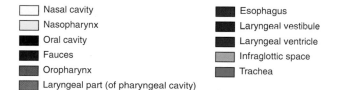

Nasal cavity		Esophagus
Nasopharynx		Laryngeal vestibule
Oral cavity		Laryngeal ventricle
Fauces		Infraglottic space
Oropharynx		Trachea
Laryngeal part (of pharyngeal cavity)		

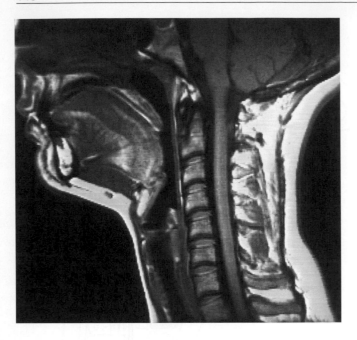

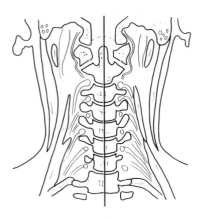

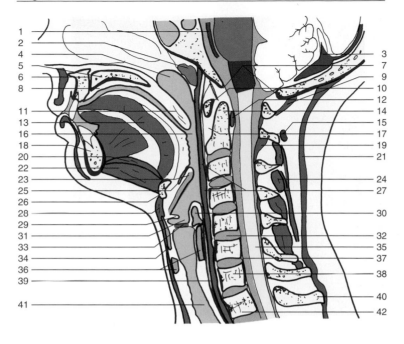

1 Basilar artery
2 Pharyngeal tonsil
3 Confluence of sinuses
4 Nasopharynx
5 Hard palate
6 Incisive fossa
7 Occipital foramen
8 Soft palate
9 Posterior atlantooccipital membrane
10 Atlas (anterior arch)
11 Uvula
12 Transverse ligament of atlas
13 Genioglossus muscle
14 Odontoid process of axis
15 Deep occipital veins
16 Oropharynx
17 Retropharyngeal space
18 Mandible
19 Flaval ligament
20 Geniohyoid muscle
21 Nuchal ligament

22 Mylohyoid muscle
23 Epiglottis
24 Interspinal muscle
25 Vallecula
26 Hyoid bone
27 Middle constrictor muscle of pharynx
28 Sternohyoid and sternothyroid muscles
29 Vestibular fold
30 Arytenoid muscle
31 Larynx (vestibule)
32 Intervertebral disk
33 Vocal cord
34 Thyroid cartilage
35 Spinal cord
36 Cricoid cartilage
37 Posterior longitudinal ligament
38 Cervical vertebra 7
39 Esophagus
40 Spinous process C7
41 Trachea
42 Anterior longitudinal ligament

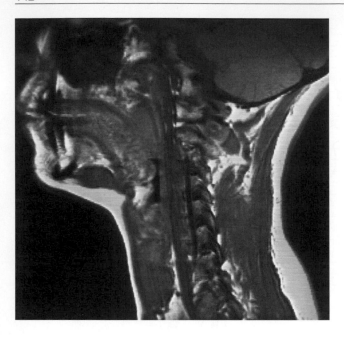

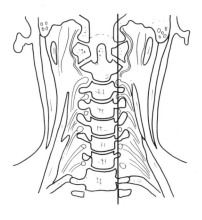

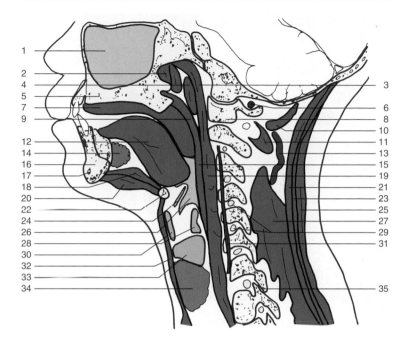

1 Maxillary sinus
2 Medial pterygoid muscle
3 Longus capitis muscle
4 Levator veli palatini muscle
5 Maxillary bone
6 Vertebral artery
7 Soft palate
8 Atlas
9 Buccinator muscle, superior constrictor muscle of pharynx
10 Rectus capitis posterior muscle (major and minor)
11 Obliquus capitis inferior muscle
12 Genioglossus muscle
13 Deep cervical vein
14 Sublingual gland
15 Middle constrictor muscle of pharynx
16 Mandible
17 Inferior alveolar artery
18 Mylohyoid muscle
19 Longus colli muscle
20 Digastric muscle (anterior belly)
21 Semispinalis capitis muscle
22 Hyoid bone
23 Splenius capitis muscle
24 Epiglottis
25 Trapezius muscle
26 Hypopharynx
27 Semispinalis cervicis muscle
28 Arytenoid cartilage
29 Nerve roots
30 Thyroid cartilage
31 Vertebral artery
32 Sternohyoid and thyrohyoid muscles
33 Cricoid cartilage
34 Thyroid gland
35 Articular facet

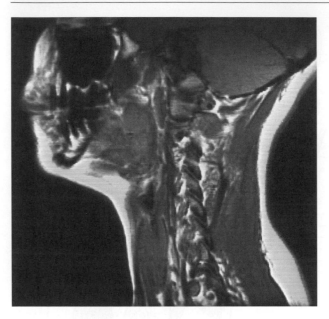

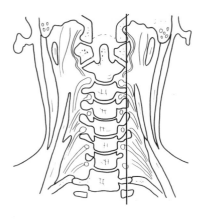

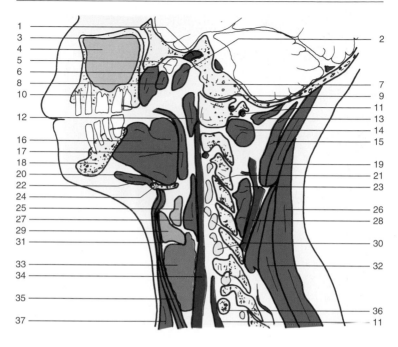

1 Internal carotid artery
2 Levator veli palatini muscle
3 Pterygopalatine fossa
4 Maxillary sinus
5 Auditory tube
6 Medial pterygoid muscle
7 Occipital condyle
8 Tensor veli palatini muscle
9 Atlantooccipital articulation
10 Maxillary bone
11 Vertebral artery
12 Longus capitis muscle
13 Rectus capitis posterior muscle (major)
14 Obliquus capitis inferior muscle
15 Semispinalis capitis muscle
16 Tongue
17 Buccinator muscle and superior
    constrictor muscle of pharynx
18 Mandible

19 Splenius capitis muscle
20 Mylohyoid muscle
21 Articular facet
22 Digastric muscle (anterior belly)
23 Multifidus muscles
24 Hyoid bone
25 Piriform sinus
26 Trapezius muscle
27 Inferior constrictor muscle of pharynx
28   Deep cervical vein
29 Thyroid cartilage
30 Nerve roots
31 Sternohyoid muscle
32 Semispinalis capitis muscle
33 Thyroid gland
34 Common carotid artery
35 Sternohyoid muscle
36 First rib
37 Sternocleidomastoid muscle

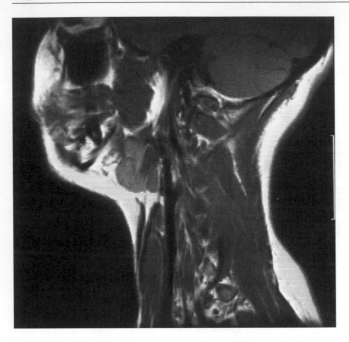

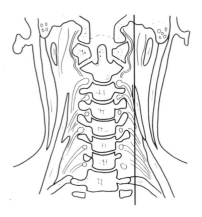

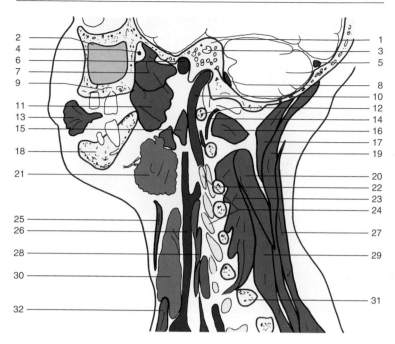

1 Temporal bone
2 Maxillary sinus
3 Cochlea
4 Maxillary artery
5 Transverse sinus
6 Internal carotid artery
7 Lateral pterygoid muscle
8 Sigmoid sinus
9 Maxillary bone
10 Internal jugular vein
11 Medial pterygoid muscle
12 Atlas (transverse process)
13 Buccinator muscle
14 Vertebral artery
15 Stylopharyngeus muscle
16 Obliquus capitis inferior muscle

17 Semispinalis capitis muscle
18 Mandible
19 Splenius capitis muscle
20 Semispinalis cervicis muscle
21 Submandibular gland
22 Transverse process
23 Multifidus muscles
24 Cervical plexus
25 Platysma
26 Common carotid artery
27 Trapezius muscle
28 Longus colli muscle
29 Splenius cervicis muscle
30 Thyroid gland
31 Rib
32 Sternocleidomastoid muscle

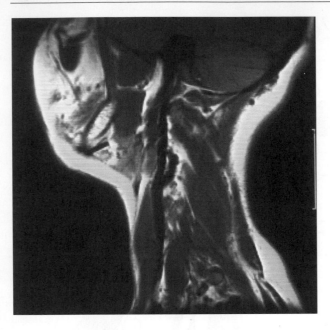

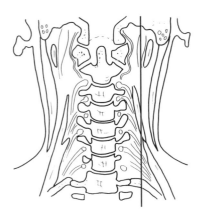

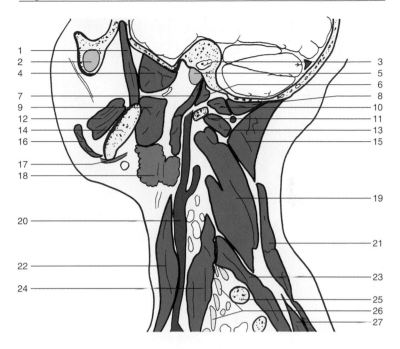

1 Temporal muscle
2 Maxillary sinus
3 Mastoid antrum
4 Lateral pterygoid muscle
5 External auditory canal
6 Rectus capitis lateralis muscle
7 Stylopharyngeus muscle
8 Rectus capitis posterior muscle (major)
9 Medial pterygoid muscle
10 Obliquus capitis inferior muscle
11 Atlas (transverse process)
12 Buccinator muscle
13 Obliquus capitis inferior muscle
14 Mandible

15 Splenius capitis muscle
16 Orbicularis oris muscle
17 Parotid duct
18 Submandibular gland
19 Multifidus muscles
20 Jugular vein
21 Trapezius muscle
22 Sternocleidomastoid muscle
23 Longus capitis muscle
24 Anterior scalene muscle
25 First rib
26 Cervical plexus
27 Levator scapulae muscle

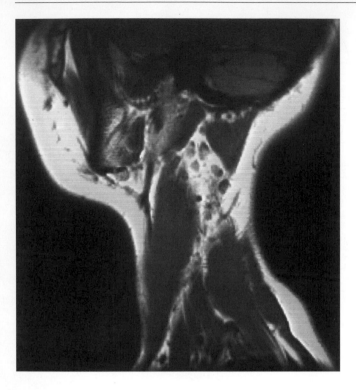

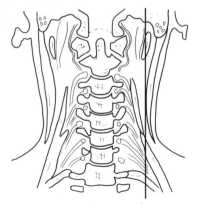

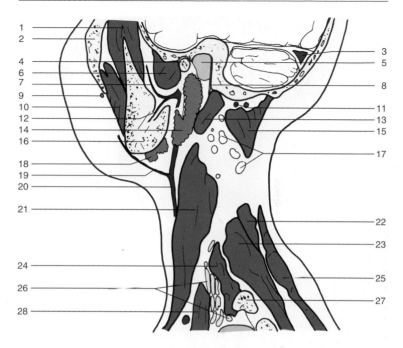

1 Temporal muscle
2 Zygomatic bone
3 Transverse sinus
4 Temporomandibular joint
5 External auditory canal
6 Lateral pterygoid muscle
7 Maxillary artery
8 Facial nerve
9 Parotid duct
10 Masseter muscle
11 Suboccipital veins
12 Inferior alveolar artery
13 Digastric muscle (posterior belly)
14 Parotid gland
15 Splenius capitis muscle
16 Mandible
17 Lymph nodes
18 Submandibular gland
19 Facial artery
20 External carotid artery
21 Sternocleidomastoid muscle
22 Longus capitis muscle
23 Levator scapulae muscle
24 Medial scalene muscle
25 Trapezius muscle
26 Brachial plexus (trunks)
27 First rib
28 Anterior scalene muscle

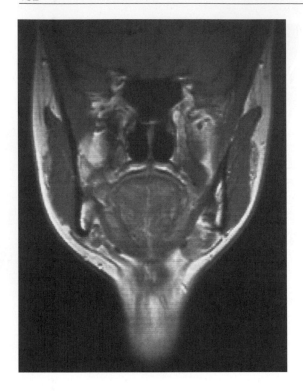

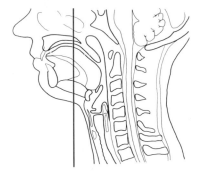

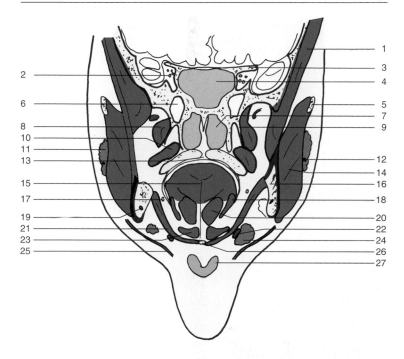

1 Temporal muscle
2 Superior orbital fissure (with optic,
trochlear, oculomotor, ophthalmic,
and abducens nerves)
3 Sphenoid bone
4 Sphenoid sinus
5 Zygomatic arch
6 Pterygopalatine fossa
7 Nasal cavity
8 Lateral pterygoid muscle
9 Pterygoid process
10 Medial pterygoid muscle
11 Parotid gland
12 Parotid duct
13 Soft palate

14 Masseter muscle
15 Tongue
16 Mandible (ramus)
17 Lingual nerve
18 Hyoglossus muscle
19 Mandibular canal (with inferior
alveolar artery, nerve, and vein)
20 Genioglossus muscle
21 Mylohyoid muscle
22 Digastric muscle (intervening tendon)
23 Geniohyoid muscle
24 Submandibular gland
25 Platysma
26 Hyoid bone
27 Thyroid cartilage

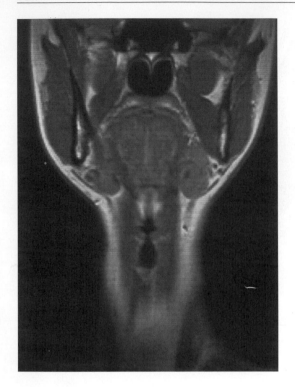

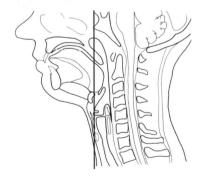

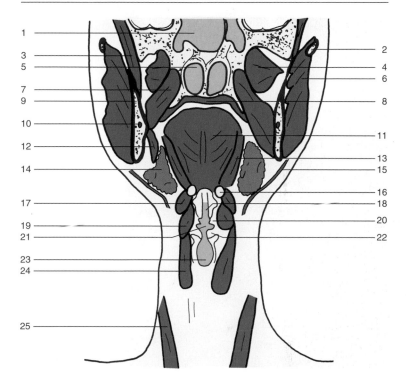

1 Sphenoid sinus
2 Zygomatic arch
3 Temporal muscle
4 Lateral pterygoid muscle
5 Nasal cavity
6 Masseter muscle
7 Medial pterygoid muscle
8 Soft palate
9 Mandible (ramus)
10 Mandibular canal
11 Tongue
12 Mylohyoid muscle
13 Hyoglossus muscle
14 Submandibular gland
15 Platysma
16 Hyoid bone
17 Omohyoid muscle
18 Preepiglottic space
19 Thyrohyoid muscle
20 Vestibular ligament
21 Laryngeal ventricle
22 Vocal ligament
23 Infraglottic cavity
24 Sternohyoid muscle
25 Sternocleidomastoid muscle

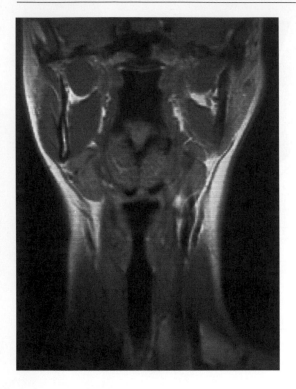

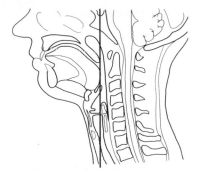

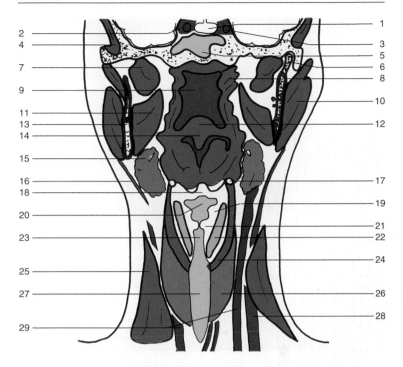

1 Pituitary gland
2 Cavernous sinus
3 Internal carotid artery
4 Temporal muscle
5 Sphenoid sinus
6 Mandible (articular condyle)
7 Lateral pterygoid muscle
8 Pharyngeal musculature
9 Nasopharynx
10 Masseter muscle
11 Medial pterygoid muscle
12 Soft palate
13 Mandible (ramus)
14 Uvula
15 Submandibular gland
16 Platysma
17 Hyoid bone (greater horn)
18 Epiglottis
19 Vestibular fold
20 Laryngeal vestibule
21 Vocal cord
22 Thyroid cartilage
23 Laryngeal cavity
24 Omohyoid, sternohyoid, and
   thyrohyoid muscles
25 Sternocleidomastoid muscle
26 Thyroid gland
27 Trachea
28 Jugular vein
29 Common carotid artery

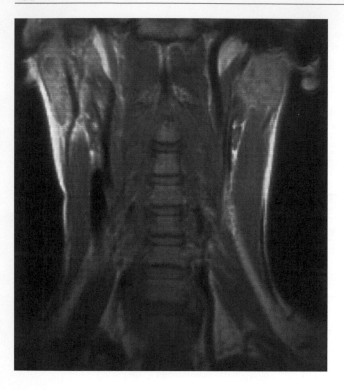

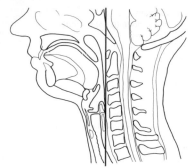

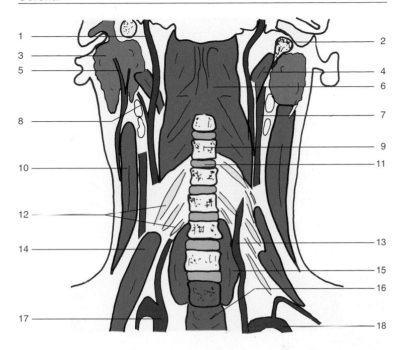

1 Internal carotid artery
2 Mandible (articular condyle)
3 Parotid gland
4 Lateral pterygoid muscle
5 Retromandibular vein
6 Constrictor muscle of pharynx
  and longus capitis muscle
7 Internal jugular vein
8 External carotid artery
9 Cervical vertebra

10 Sternocleidomastoid muscle
11 Intervertebral disk
12 Cervical plexus
13 Vertebral artery
14 Anterior scalene muscle
15 Longissimus cervicis muscle
16 Esophagus
17 Brachiocephalic trunk
18 Subclavian artery

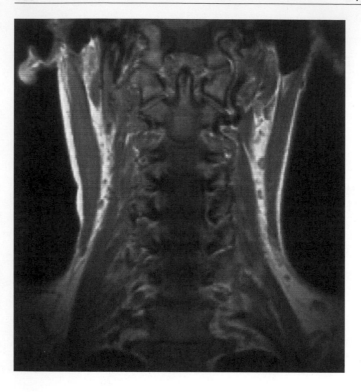

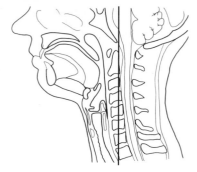

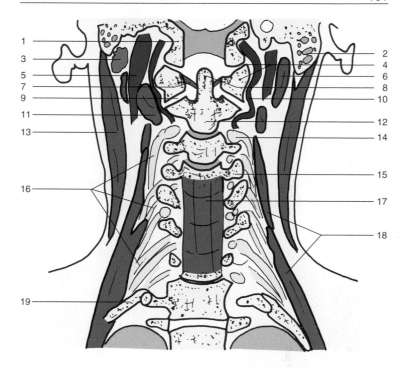

1 Occipital condyle
2 Mastoid process
3 Parotid gland
4 Atlas (lateral mass) and
   atlantooccipital articulation
5 Jugular vein
6 Digastric muscle
7 Alar ligaments
8 Odontoid process of axis
9 Atlantoaxial articulation
10 Vertebral artery

11 Obliquus inferior muscle
12 Axis
13 Sternocleidomastoid muscle
14 Root of nerve C3
15 Transverse process C4
16 Cervical plexus (trunks)
17 Posterior longitudinal ligament
   (and cervical vertebrae)
18 Medial and posterior scalene muscles
19 First rib

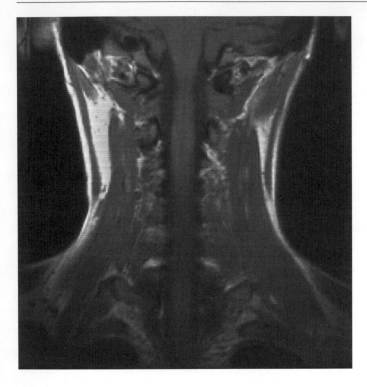

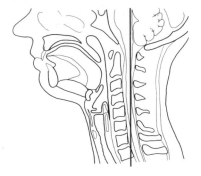

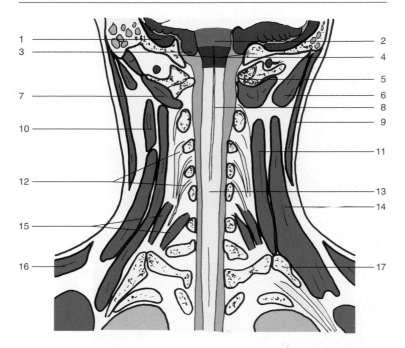

1 Sigmoid sinus
2 Pons and medulla oblongata
3 Tonsil of Cerebellum
4 Occipital foramen
5 Atlas
6 Splenius cervicis muscle
7 Obliquus inferior muscle
8 Median fissure (central canal)
9 Sternocleidomastoid muscle
10 Longissimus capitis muscle
11 Semispinalis cervicis muscle
12 Cervical plexus
13 Spinal cord
14 Levator scapulae muscle
15 Multifidus muscles
16 Trapezius muscle
17 First rib

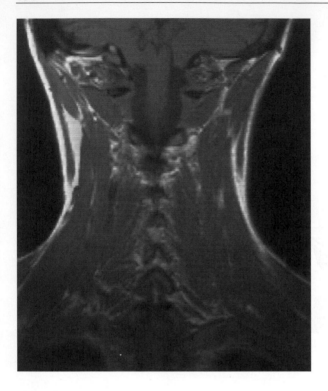

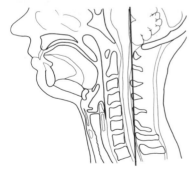

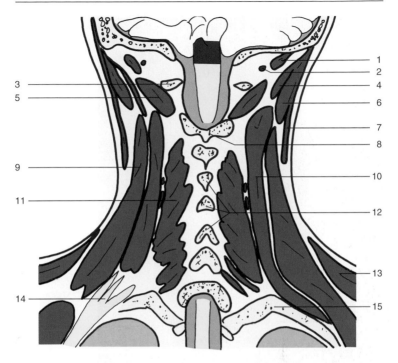

1 Obliquus capitis superior muscle
2 Deep cervical vein
3 Transverse process of cervical vertebra 1
4 Longissimus capitis muscle
5 Obliquus inferior muscle
6 Splenius capitis muscle
7 Sternocleidomastoid muscle
8 Spinous process of axis

9 Levator scapulae muscle
10 Semispinalis muscle
11 Multifidus muscles
12 Spinous processes (cervical vertebra 4 - 6)
13 Trapezius muscle
14 Cervical plexus
15 Rib

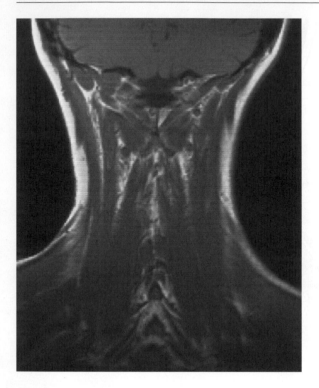

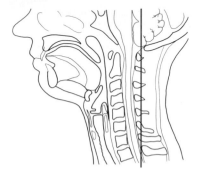

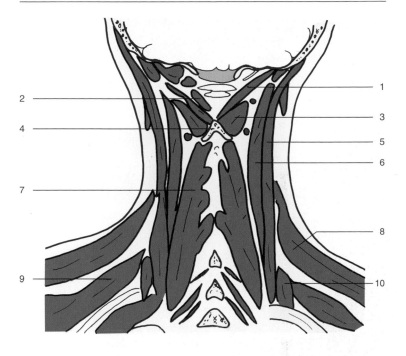

1 Rectus capitis posterior muscle (major)
2 Rectus capitis posterior muscle (minor)
3 Obliquus capitis inferior muscle
4 Spinous process of axis
5 Splenius capitis muscle

6 Semispinalis capitis muscle
7 Multifidus muscles
8 Trapezius muscle
9 Levator scapulae muscle
10 Rhomboid muscle

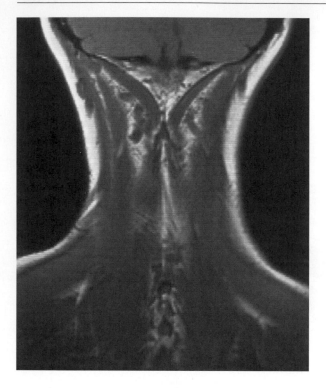

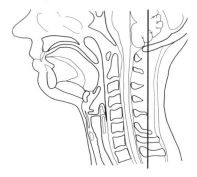

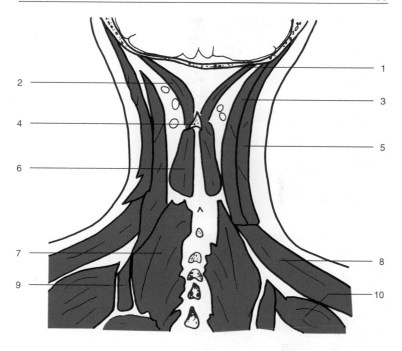

1 Occipital bone
2 Rectus capitis posterior muscle (major)
3 Semispinalis capitis muscle
4 Spinous process of axis
5 Splenius capitis muscle

6 Semispinalis cervicis muscle
7 Multifidus muscles
8 Trapezius muscle
9 Rhomboid muscle
10 Levator scapulae muscle

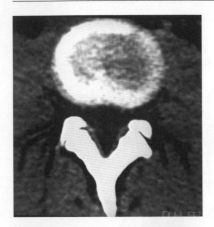

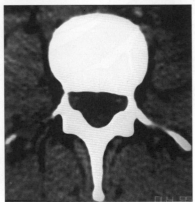

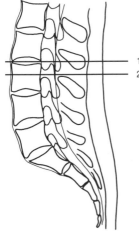

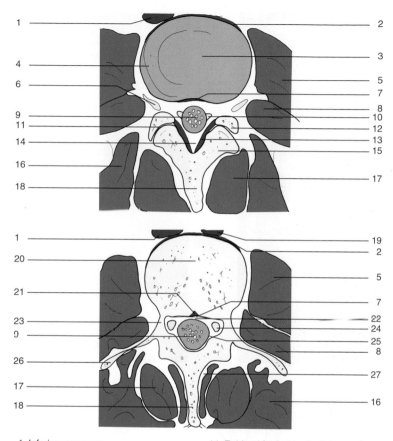

1 Inferior vena cava
2 Anterior longitudinal ligament
3 Intervertebral disk (L2/L3)
4 Anulus fibrosus
5 Psoas muscle
6 Spinal nerve L2
7 Posterior longitudinal ligament
8 Quadratus lumborum muscle
9 Cauda equina (in dural sac)
10 Spinal nerve L3 (exiting dural sac)
11 Zygapophyseal articulation
   (articular facet)
12 Superior articular process
13 Flaval ligament

14 Epidural fat (retrospinal trigonum)
15 Inferior articular process
16 Erector spinae muscle
17 Multifidus muscles
18 Spinous process
19 Aorta (bifurcation)
20 Lumbar vertebra 3
21 Basivertebral veins
22 Internal vertebral venous plexus
23 Pedicle
24 Nerve root
25 Dural sac
26 Transverse process
27 Paraspinal fat tissue

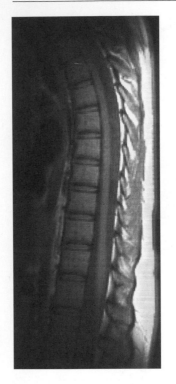
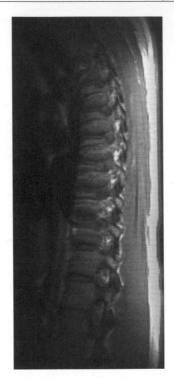

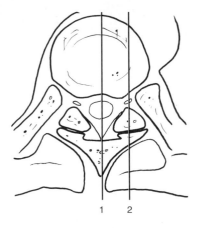

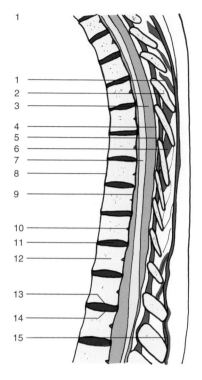
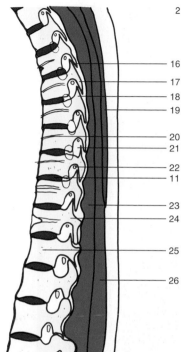

1 Supraspinal ligaments
2 Spinous process
3 Cerebrospinal fluid
   (postmedullary thecal space)
4 Epidural fat
5 Flaval ligament
6 Interspinal ligaments
7 Spinal cord
8 Anterior longitudinal ligament
9 Posterior longitudinal ligament
10 Basivertebral veins
11 Intervertebral disk
12 Thoracic vertebra
13 Inferior surface of vertebral body

14 Superior surface of vertebral body
15 Thoracolumbar fascia
16 Zygapophyseal articulation
   (articular facet)
17 Superior articular process
18 Inferior articular process
19 Trapezius muscle
20 Thoracic vessel
21 Intervertebral foramen
22 Nerve root
23 Multifidus muscles
24 Pedicle
25 Vertebral body
26 Erector spinae muscle

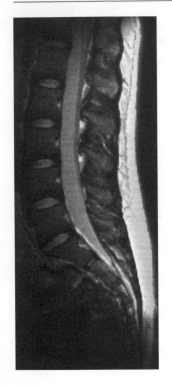
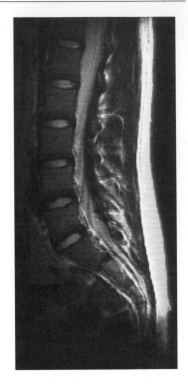

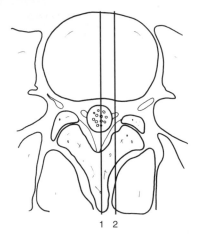

1 2

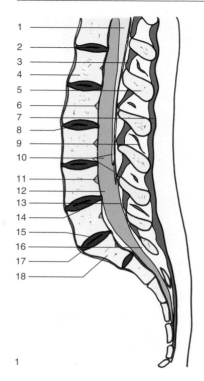
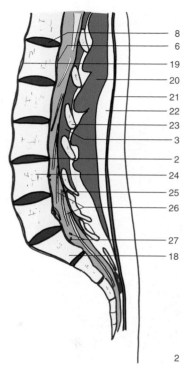

1 Conus medullaris
2 Anulus fibrosus
3 Flaval ligament
4 Lumbar vertebra 1
5 Spinous process (L1)
6 Posterior longitudinal ligament
7 Supraspinal ligaments
8 Intervertebral disk (with intranuclear cleft, MR sign of adult intervertebral disk)
9 Interspinal ligaments (with interspinal bursa)
10 Cauda equina
11 Basivertebral veins
12 Thecal sac
13 Dura

14 Superior surface of vertebral body
15 Inferior surface of vertebral body
16 Epidural fat
17 Promontory
18 Sacral vertebra 1
19 Anterior longitudinal ligament
20 Multifidus muscles
21 Lumbosacral fascia
22 Erector spinae muscle
23 Vertebral arch
24 Lumbar vertebra 4
25 Zygapophyseal articulation (articular facet)
26 Nerve roots
27 Internal vertebral venous plexus

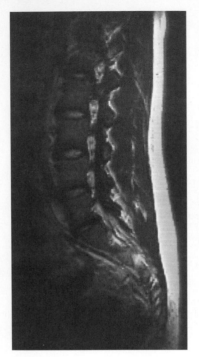
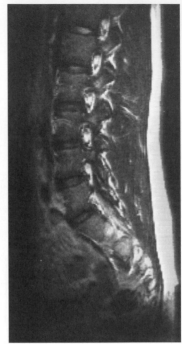
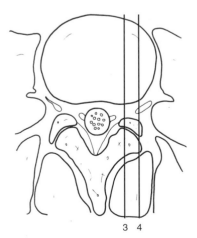

3 4

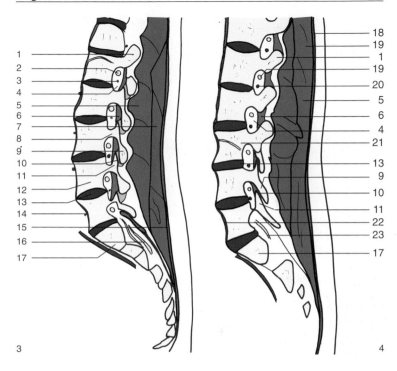

3   4

 1 Mamillary process
 2 Spinal nerve root L1
 3 Spinal branch of segmental artery
 4 Intervertebral foramen
 5 Multifidus muscles
 6 Flaval ligament
 7 Erector spinae muscle
 8 Vertebral pedicle (L3)
 9 Inferior articular process
10 Zygapophyseal articulation
    (articular facet)
11 Superior articular process

12 Lumbar vertebra 4
13 Intervertebral disk
14 Anterior longitudinal ligament
15 Lumbodorsal ligament
16 Sacral nerve roots
17 Sacral vertebra 1
18 Lumbodorsal fascia (thoracolumbar)
19 Spinal nerve L2
20 Spinal branch of segmental artery (L2)
21 Lumbar vertebra 3
22 Anterior longitudinal ligament
23 Spinal nerve S1

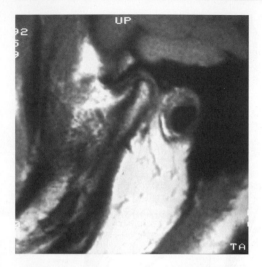

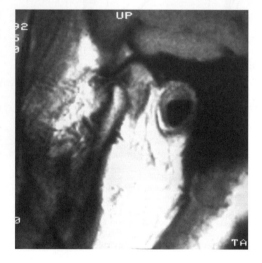

cranial
ventral ☐ dorsal
caudal

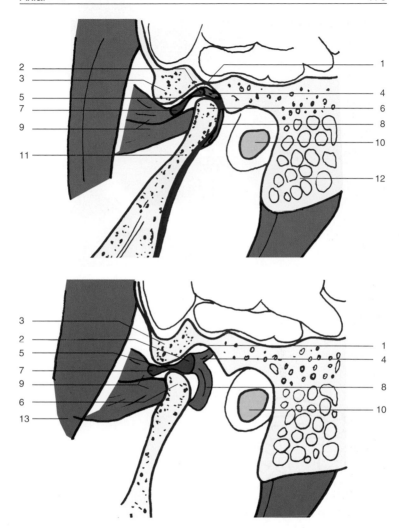

1 Mandibular fossa
2 Posterior ligament (articular disk)
3 Articular tubercle
4 Upper retrodiscal lamina of bilaminar zone
5 Intermediate zone (articular disk)
6 Condyle of mandible
7 Anterior ligament (articular disk)
8 Rear retrodiscal lamina of bilaminar zone
9 Lateral pterygoid muscle
10 External auditory canal
11 Mandibular neck
12 Mastoid air cells
13 Temporal muscle

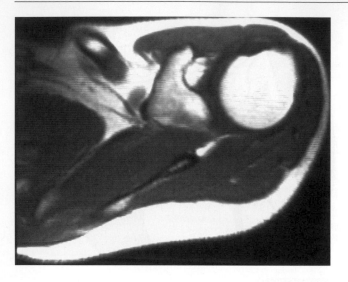

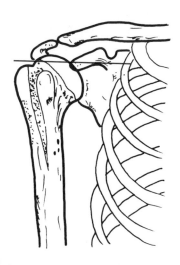

ventral

medial [ ] lateral

dorsal

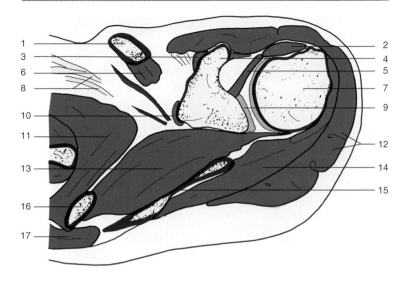

1 Clavicle
2 Supraspinatus muscle (tendon)
3 Pectoralis minor muscle (tendon)
4 Coracoid process
5 Biceps muscle (long head, tendon)
6 Subclavius muscle
7 Humerus (head)
8 Brachial plexus
9 Glenoid fossa
10 Coracoclavicular ligament
11 Serratus anterior muscle
12 Deltoid muscle
13 Supraspinatus muscle
14 Infraspinatus muscle
15 Spine of scapula
16 Rib
17 Trapezius muscle

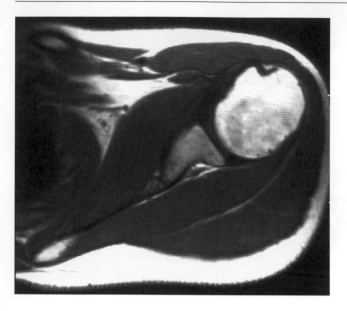

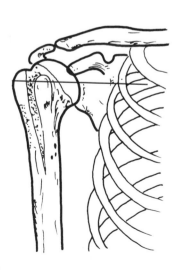

ventral

medial [ ] lateral

dorsal

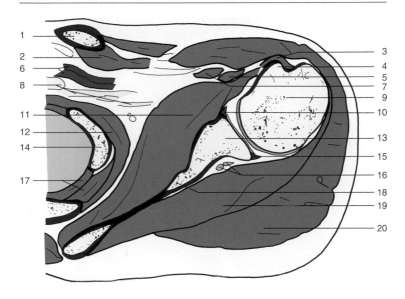

1 Clavicle
2 Subclavius muscle
3 Biceps muscle (long head, tendon)
4 Lesser tubercle
5 Biceps muscle (short head)
6 Axillary artery and vein
7 Coracobrachialis muscle
8 Brachial plexus
9 Head of humerus
10 Anterior glenoid lip

11 Subscapularis muscle
12 Serratus anterior muscle
13 Glenoid fossa
14 Rib
15 Posterior glenoid lip
16 Suprascapular artery, vein, and nerve
17 Intercostal muscles
18 Scapula
19 Teres minor muscle
20 Deltoid muscle

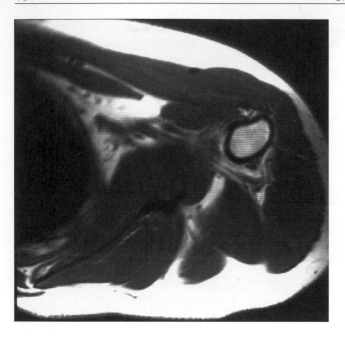

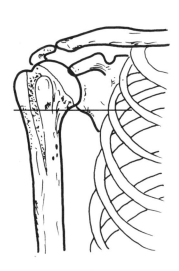

ventral

medial ☐ lateral

dorsal

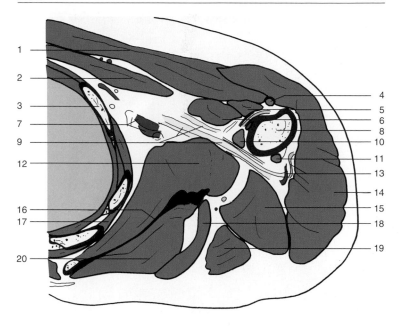

1 Pectoralis major muscle
2 Pectoralis minor muscle
3 Rib
4 Biceps muscle (long head)
5 Biceps muscle (short head)
6 Coracobrachialis muscle
7 Axillary artery and vein
8 Humerus
9 Brachial plexus
10 Subscapularis muscle

11 Triceps muscle (lateral head)
12 Subscapularis muscle
13 Posterior humeral circumflex artery and vein
14 Deltoid muscle
15 Triceps muscle (long head)
16 Scapula
17 Serratus anterior muscle
18 Teres major muscle
19 Latissimus dorsi muscle
20 Infraspinatus muscle

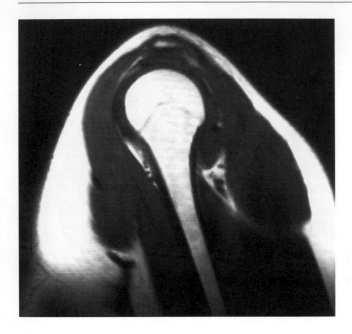

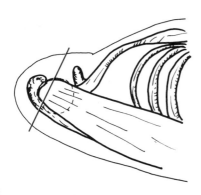

proximal

ventral ☐ dorsal

distal

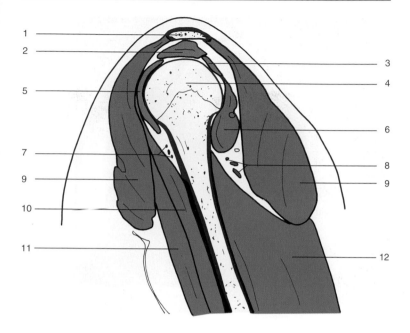

1 Acromion
2 Supraspinatus muscle (tendon)
3 Infraspinatus muscle (tendon)
4 Humerus (head)
5 Biceps muscle (long head, tendon)
6 Teres minor muscle
7 Anterior humeral circumflex artery
 and vein

8 Posterior humeral circumflex artery
 and vein
9 Deltoid muscle
10 Coracobrachialis muscle
11 Biceps muscle (short head)
12 Triceps muscle

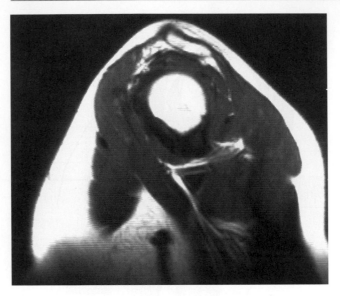

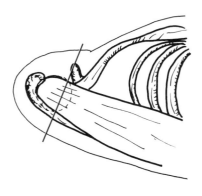

proximal

ventral ☐ dorsal

distal

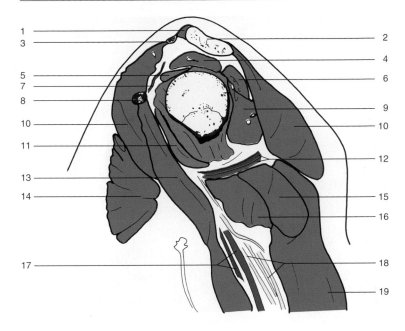

1 Trapezius muscle
2 Scapula
3 Clavicle
4 Supraspinatus muscle
5 Biceps muscle (long head, tendon)
6 Infraspinatus muscle
7 Coracoacromial ligament
8 Coracoid process
9 Teres minor muscle
10 Deltoid muscle

11 Subscapularis muscle
12 Posterior humeral circumflex artery and vein
13 Coracobrachialis muscle
14 Pectoralis major muscle
15 Teres major muscle
16 Latissimus dorsi muscle
17 Brachial artery and vein
18 Brachial plexus
19 Triceps muscle

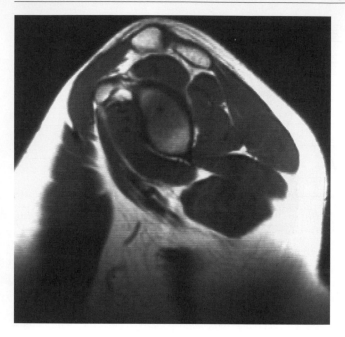

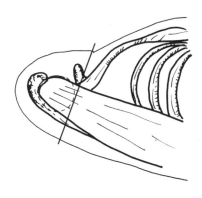

proximal

ventral ☐ dorsal

distal

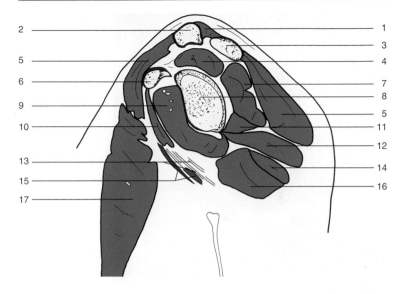

1 Trapezius muscle
2 Clavicle
3 Spine of scapula
4 Supraspinatus muscle
5 Deltoid muscle
6 Coracoid process
7 Infraspinatus muscle
8 Glenoid fossa
9 Subscapularis muscle
10 Coracobrachialis muscle
11 Teres minor muscle
12 Triceps muscle
13 Brachial plexus
14 Teres major muscle
15 Axillary artery and vein
16 Latissimus dorsi muscle
17 Pectoralis major muscle

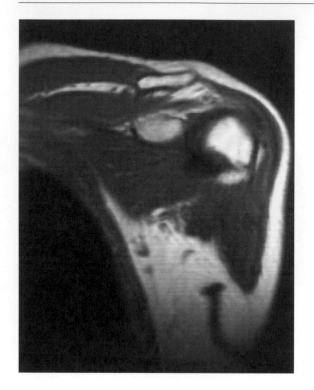

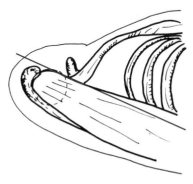

proximal

medial ☐ lateral

distal

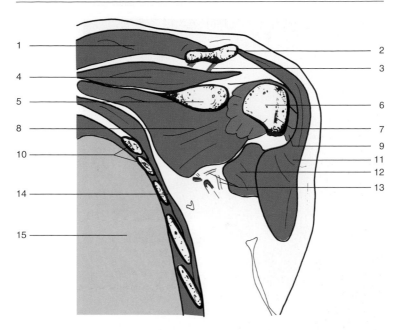

1 Trapezius muscle
2 Clavicle
3 Coracoacromial ligament
4 Supraspinatus muscle
5 Coracoid process
6 head of humerus
7 Intertubercular groove
8 Subscapularis muscle
9 Articular capsule
10 Rib
11 Deltoid muscle
12 Coracobrachialis muscle
13 Brachial plexus
14 Serratus anterior muscle
15 Lung

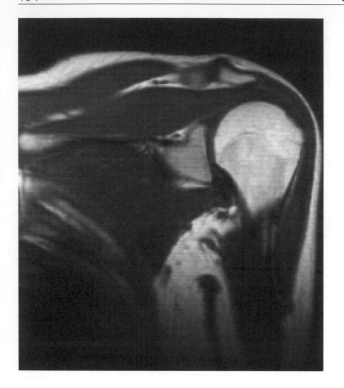

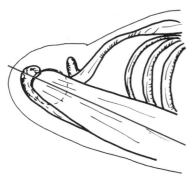

proximal

medial ☐ lateral

distal

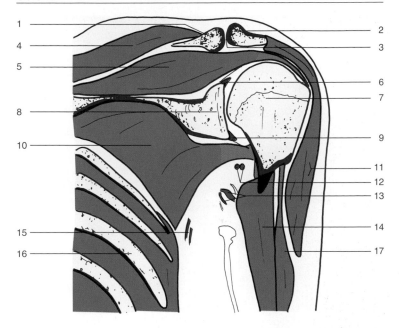

1 Clavicle
2 Acromion
3 Acromioclavicular joint
4 Trapezius muscle
5 Supraspinatus muscle
6 Superior glenoid lip
7 Head of humerus
8 Glenoid fossa (scapula)
9 Inferior glenoid lip

10 Subscapularis muscle
11 Deltoid muscle
12 Posterior humeral circumflex artery
13 Axillary artery and vein
14 Coracobrachialis muscle
15 Subscapularis artery, vein, and nerve
16 Ribs
17 Biceps muscle (long head)

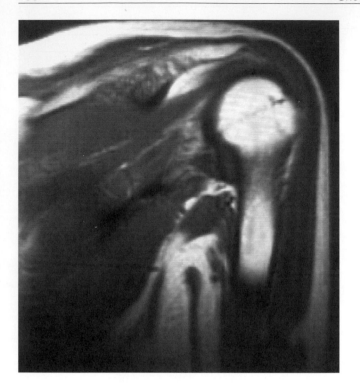

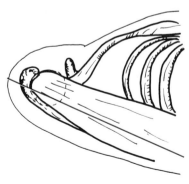

proximal

medial ☐ lateral

distal

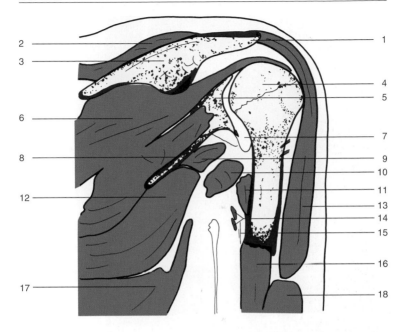

1 Acromion
2 Trapezius muscle
3 Spine of scapula
4 Head of humerus
5 Glenoid fossa
6 Infraspinatus muscle
7 Axillar recess
8 Scapula
9 Teres minor muscle

10 Latissimus dorsi muscle
11 Triceps muscle
12 Teres major muscle
13 Deltoid muscle
14 Brachial artery and vein
15 Median nerve
16 Coracobrachialis muscle
17 Latissimus dorsi muscle
18 Biceps muscle

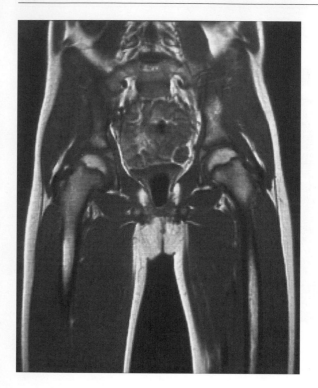

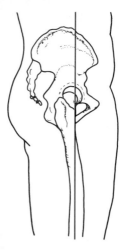

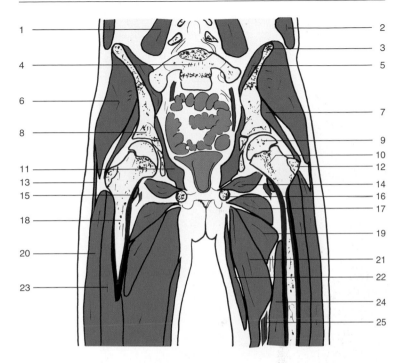

1 Psoas muscle
2 Internal oblique muscle
3 Ilium
4 Sacrum
5 Iliac muscle
6 Gluteus medius muscle
7 Gluteus minimus muscle
8 Acetabulum (ilium)
9 Head of femur
10 Neck of femur
11 Internal obturator muscle
12 Greater trochanter
13 Iliotibial tract

14 External obturator muscle
15 Iliopsoas muscle
16 Pubis (inferior ramus)
17 Adductor brevis muscle
18 Femur
19 Adductor longus muscle
20 Vastus lateralis muscle
21 Adductor magnus muscle
22 Gracilis muscle
23 Vastus intermedius muscle
24 Vastus medialis muscle
25 Femoral artery and vein

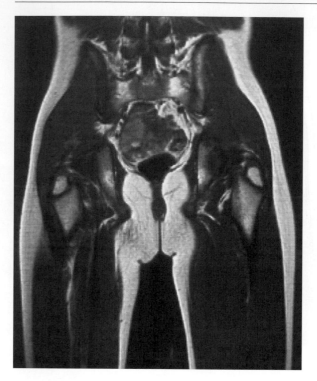

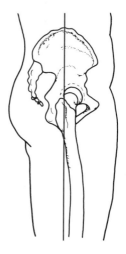

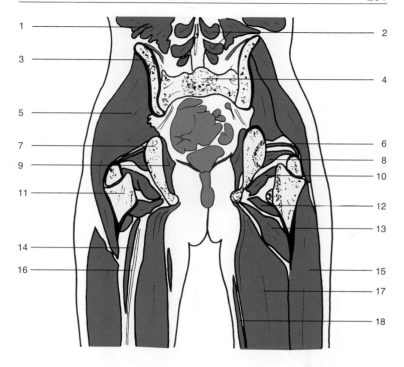

1 Quadratus lumborum muscle
2 Multifidus muscles
3 Ilium
4 Sacrum
5 Gluteus medius muscle
6 Gemellus muscles (tendon)
7 Ischium
8 External obturator muscle
9 Internal obturator muscle
10 Quadratus femoris muscle
11 Femur
12 Adductor brevis muscle
13 Adductor longus muscle
14 Biceps femoris muscle
15 Vastus lateralis muscle
16 Sciatic nerve
17 Adductor magnus muscle
18 Gracilis muscle

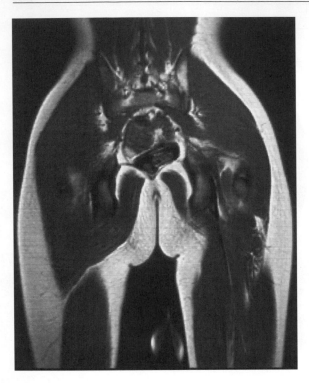

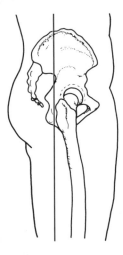

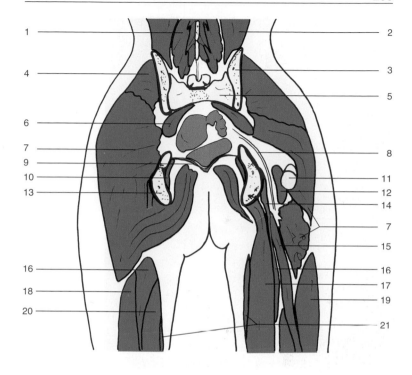

1 Multifidus muscles
2 Quadratus lumborum muscle
3 Ilium
4 Gluteus medius muscle
5 Sacrum (ala)
6 Piriform muscle
7 Gluteus maximus muscle
8 Sciatic nerve
9 Levator ani muscle
10 Internal obturator muscle
11 Greater trochanter

12 Piriform muscle
13 Ischial tuberosity
14 Semitendinosus muscle
15 Biceps femoris muscle (long head)
16 Semitendinosus muscle
17 Adductor magnus muscle
18 Biceps femoris muscle (short head)
19 Vastus lateralis muscle
20 Semimembranosus muscle
21 Gracilis muscle

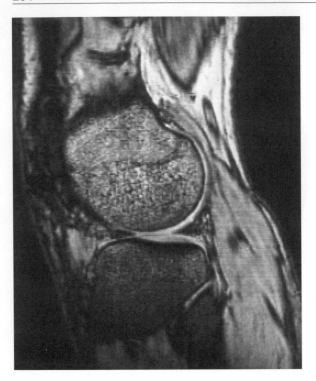

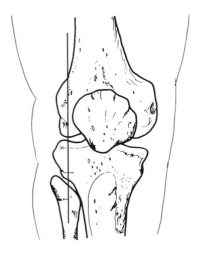

proximal

ventral ☐ dorsal

distal

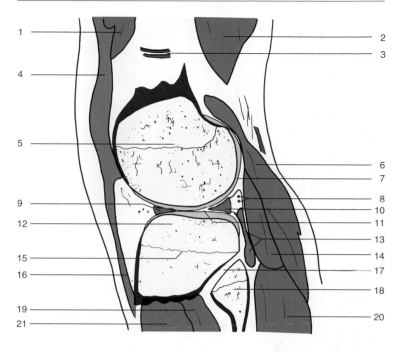

1 Vastus lateralis muscle
2 Biceps femoris muscle
3 Lateral superior genicular artery
4 Lateral patellar retinaculum
5 Lateral condyle of femur
6 Gastrocnemius muscle (lateral head)
7 Articular cartilage
8 Lateral inferior genicular artery
9 Lateral meniscus (anterior horn)
10 Lateral meniscus (posterior horn)
11 Joint space

12 Lateral condyle of tibia
13 Popliteal muscle (tendon)
14 Plantar muscle
15 Epiphyseal line
16 Patellar ligament
17 Tibiofibular articulation
18 Fibula
19 Extensor digitorum longus muscle
20 Soleus muscle
21 Tibialis anterior muscle

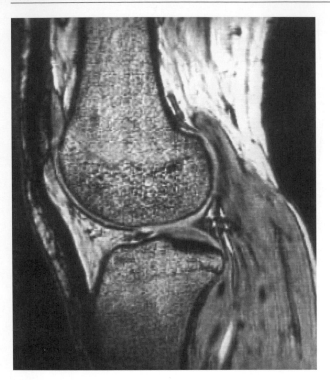

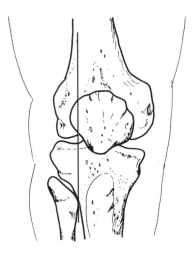

proximal

ventral [ ] dorsal

distal

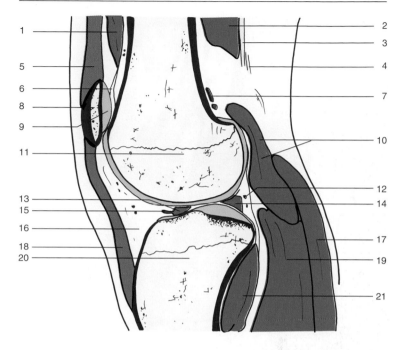

1 Vastus intermedius muscle
2 Biceps femoris muscle
3 Common peroneal nerve
4 Tibial nerve
5 Quadriceps femoris muscle (tendon)
6 Suprapatellar bursa
7 Lateral superior genicular artery
8 Patella
9 Retropatellar cartilage
10 Plantar muscle
11 Lateral femur condyle

12 Lateral inferior genicular artery
13 Lateral meniscus (anterior horn)
14 Lateral meniscus (posterior horn)
15 Transverse ligament of knee
16 Infrapatellar fat pad
17 Gastrocnemius muscle (lateral head)
18 Patellar ligament
19 Soleus muscle
20 Tibia
21 Popliteal muscle

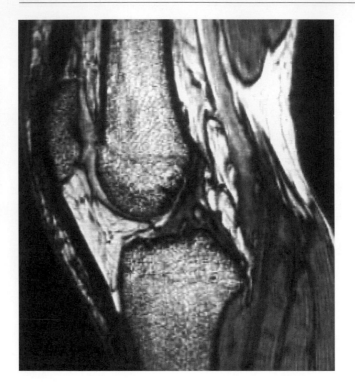

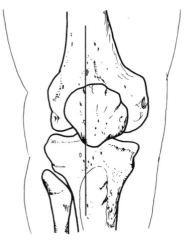

proximal

ventral [ ] dorsal

distal

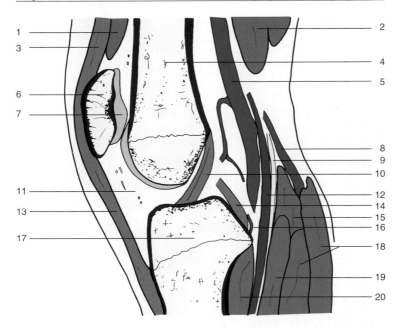

1 Vastus medialis muscle
2 Semimembranosus muscle
3 Rectus femoris muscle (tendon)
4 Femur
5 Femoral vein
6 Patella
7 Retropatellar cartilage
8 Small saphenous vein
9 Tibialis nerve
10 Anterior cruciate ligament
11 Infrapatellar fat pad
12 Popliteal artery
13 Patellar ligament
14 Posterior cruciate ligament
15 Gastrocnemius muscle (medial head)
16 Meniscofemoral ligament
17 Tibia
18 Gastrocnemius muscle (lateral head)
19 Soleus muscle
20 Popliteal muscle

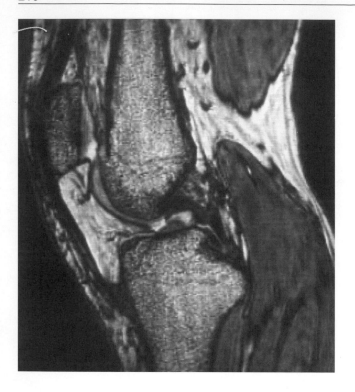

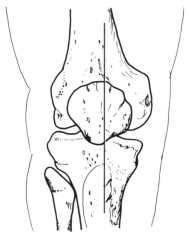

proximal

ventral ☐ dorsal

distal

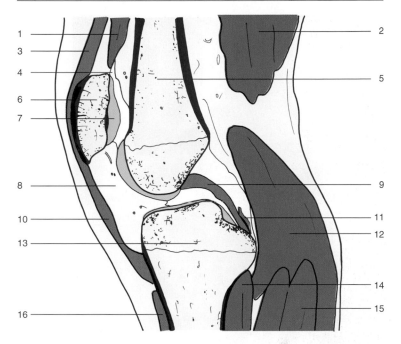

1 Vastus medialis muscle
2 Semimembranosus muscle
3 Quadriceps femoris muscle (tendon)
4 Suprapatellar bursa
5 Femur
6 Patella
7 Retropatellar cartilage
8 Infrapatellar fat pad

9 Posterior cruciate ligament
10 Patellar ligament
11 Meniscofemoral ligament
12 Gastrocnemius muscle
13 Tibia
14 Popliteal muscle
15 Soleus muscle
16 Tibialis anterior muscle

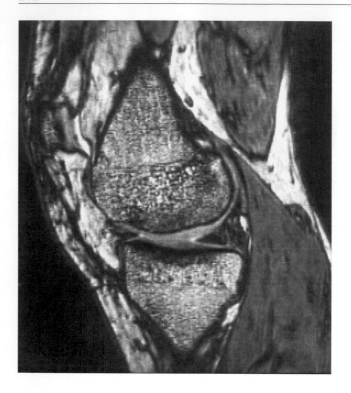

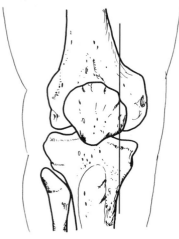

proximal

ventral [ ] dorsal

distal

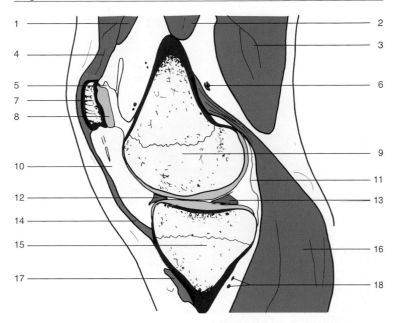

1 Vastus medialis muscle
2 Sartorius muscle
3 Semimembranosus muscle
4 Quadriceps femoris muscle (tendon)
5 Suprapatellar bursa
6 Medial superior genicular artery and vein
7 Patella
8 Retropatellar cartilage
9 Medial condyle of femur
10 Infrapatellar fat pad
11 Joint capsule
12 Medial meniscus (anterior horn)
13 Medial meniscus (posterior horn)
14 Patellar ligament
15 Medial condyle of tibia
16 Gastrocnemius muscle (medial head)
17 Sartorius muscle (insertion of tendon)
18 Medial inferior genicular artery and vein

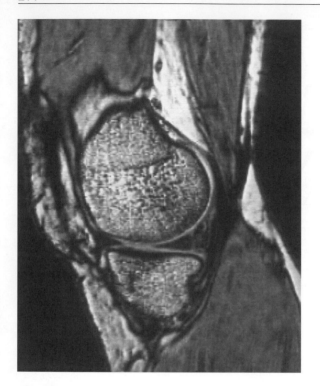

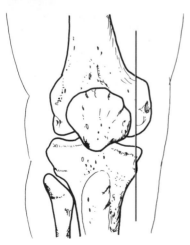

proximal

ventral ☐ dorsal

distal

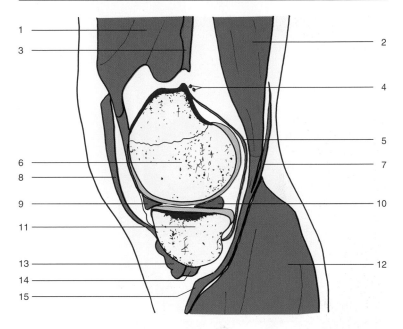

1 Vastus medialis muscle
2 Semimembranosus muscle
3 Adductor magnus muscle
4 Medial superior genicular artery and vein
5 Joint capsule
6 Medial condyle of femur
7 Semitendinosus muscle (tendon)
8 Medial patellar retinaculum

9 Medial meniscus (anterior horn)
10 Medial meniscus (posterior horn)
11 Tibia
12 Gastrocnemius muscle (medial head)
13 Sartorius muscle (insertion of tendon)
14 Gracilis muscle (insertion of tendon)
15 Pes anserinus

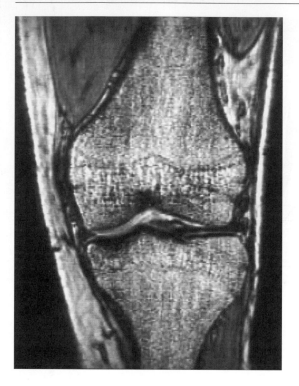

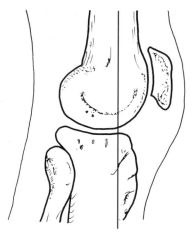

proximal

medial ☐ lateral

distal

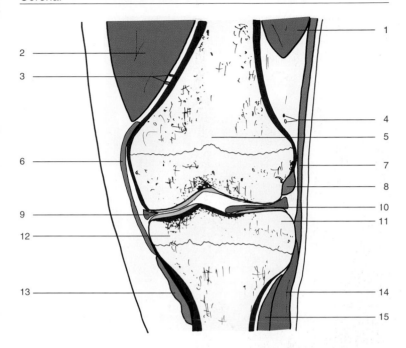

1 Vastus lateralis muscle
2 Vastus medialis muscle
3 Medial superior genicular artery
4 Lateral superior genicular artery
5 Femur
6 Tibial collateral ligament
7 Iliotibial tract
8 Popliteal muscle (tendon)
9 Medial meniscus
10 Lateral meniscus (anterior horn)
11 Lateral tibia plateau
12 Medial tibia plateau
13 Pes anserinus
14 Peroneus longus muscle
15 Extensor digitorum longus muscle

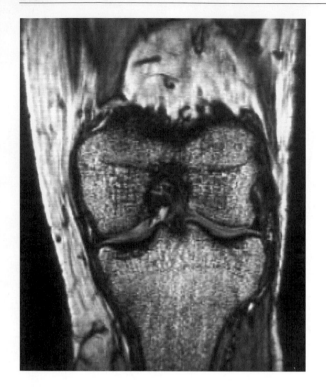

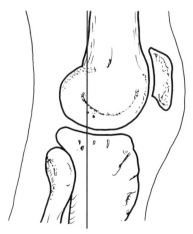

proximal

medial ☐ lateral

distal

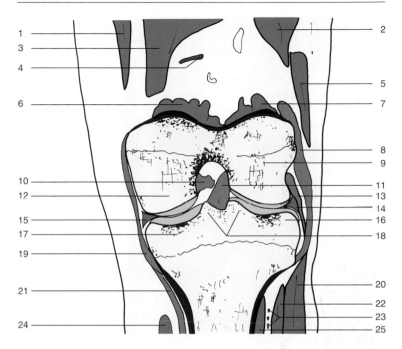

1 Sartorius muscle
2 Vastus lateralis muscle
3 Semimembranosus muscle
4 Medial superior genicular artery
5 Biceps femoris muscle
6 Gastrocnemius muscle (medial head)
7 Gastrocnemius muscle (lateral head)
8 Iliotibial tract
9 Lateral condyle of femur
10 Posterior cruciate ligament
11 Anterior cruciate ligament
12 Medial condyle of femur
13 Popliteal muscle (tendon)

14 Lateral meniscus
15 Medial meniscus
16 Lateral tibia plateau
17 Medial tibia plateau
18 Intercondylar eminence
19 Tibial collateral ligament
20 Peroneus longus muscle
21 Gracilis muscle (tendon)
22 Extensor digitorum longus muscle
23 Lateral inferior genicular artery and vein
24 Semitendinosus muscle (tendon)
25 Tibialis posterior muscle

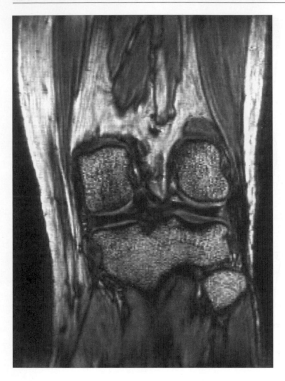

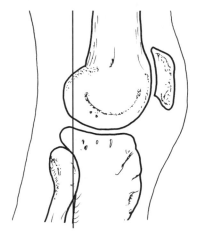

proximal

medial ☐ lateral

distal

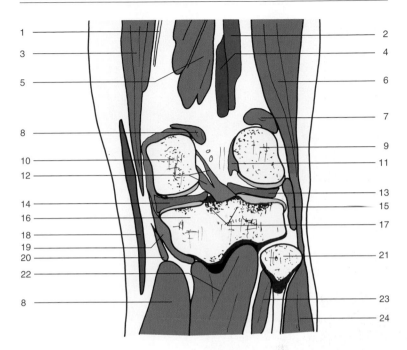

1 Saphenous nerve
3 Sartorius muscle
5 Semimembranosus muscle
8 Gastrocnemius muscle (medial head)

1 Saphenous nerve
2 Popliteal vein
3 Sartorius muscle
4 Popliteal artery
5 Semimembranosus muscle
6 Biceps femoris muscle
7 Gastrocnemius muscle (lateral head)
8 Gastrocnemius muscle (medial head)
9 Lateral condyle of femur
10 Medial condyle of femur
11 Anterior cruciate ligament
12 Posterior cruciate ligament

13 Lateral meniscus
14 Medial meniscus
15 Popliteal muscle (tendon)
16 Medial condyle of tibia
17 Intercondylar eminence
18 Great saphenous vein
19 Semimembranosus muscle
20 Gracilis muscle (tendon)
21 Head of fibula
22 Popliteal muscle
23 Tibialis posterior muscle
24 Peroneus longus muscle

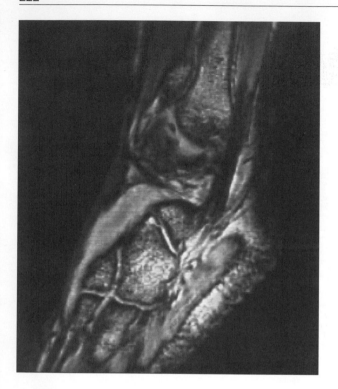

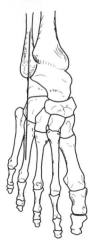

proximal
dorsal

anterior [ ] posterior

plantar
distal

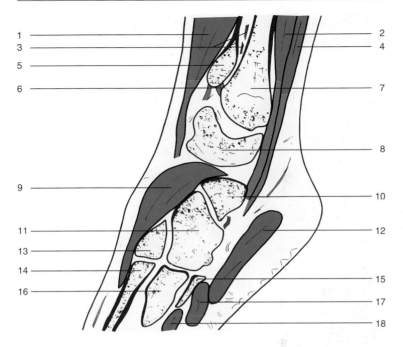

1 Extensor digitorum longus muscle
2 Peroneus longus muscle
3 Tibialis anterior artery and vein
4 Peroneus brevis muscle
5 Tibia
6 Anterior tibiofibular ligament
7 Fibula (lateral malleolus)
8 Talus
9 Extensor digitorum brevis muscle
10 Calcaneus
11 Cuboid bone
12 Abductor digiti minimi muscle
13 Lateral cuneiform bone
14 Metatarsal bone III
15 Metatarsal bone V
16 Metatarsal bone IV
17 Flexor digiti minimi brevis muscle
18 Interosseous muscle

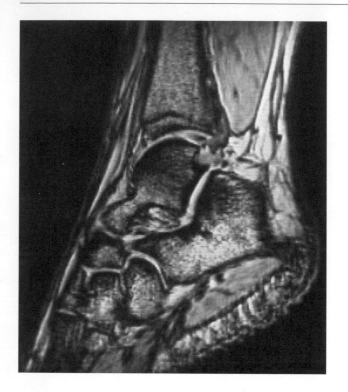

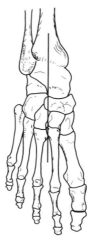

proximal
dorsal

anterior ☐ posterior

plantar
distal

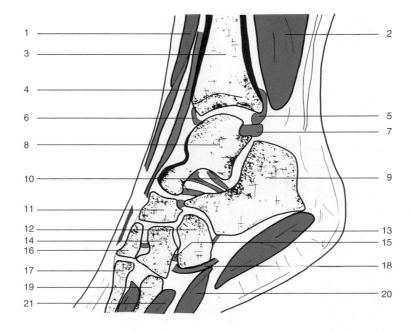

1 Extensor hallucis longus muscle
2 Flexor hallucis longus muscle
3 Tibia
4 Extensor digitorum longus muscle
  (tendon)
5 Posterior tibiofibular ligament
6 Joint capsule
7 Posterior tibiofibular ligament
8 Talus
9 Calcaneus
10 Interosseous talocalcaneal ligament

11 Navicular bone
12 Cuboid bone
13 Abductor digiti minimi muscle
14 Lateral cuneiform bone
15 Interosseous ligament
16 Medial cuneiform bone
17 Metatarsal bone II
18 Peroneus longus muscle (tendon)
19 Metatarsal bone III
20 Opponens digiti minimi muscle
21 Lumbrical and interosseous muscles

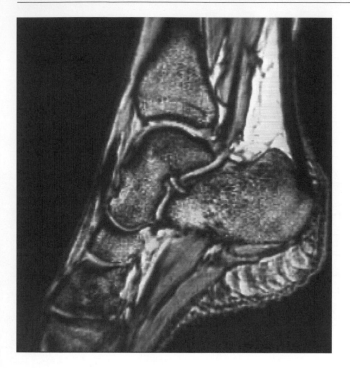

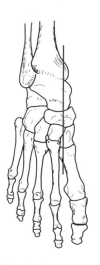

proximal
dorsal

anterior [ ] posterior

plantar
distal

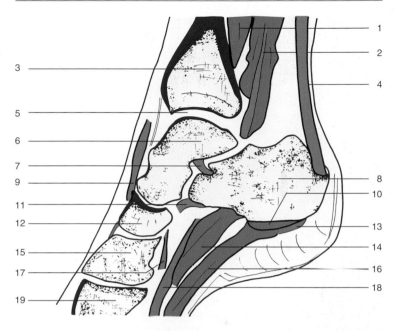

1 Tibialis posterior muscle
2 Flexor hallucis longus muscle
3 Tibia
4 Achilles tendon
5 Talocrural joint
6 Talus
7 Interosseous talocalcaneal ligament
8 Calcaneus
9 Tibialis anterior muscle (tendon)
10 Abductor digiti minimi muscle

11 Plantar calcaneonavicular ligament
12 Navicular bone
13 Plantar aponeurosis
14 Quadratus plantae muscle
15 Intermediate cuneiform bone
16 Flexor digitorum brevis muscle
17 Tibialis posterior muscle (tendon)
18 Flexor digitorum longus muscle (tendon)
19 Metatarsal bone II (base)

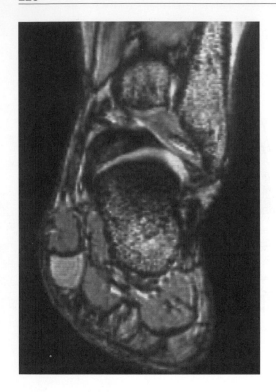

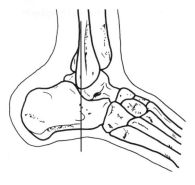

proximal

medial ☐ lateral

distal

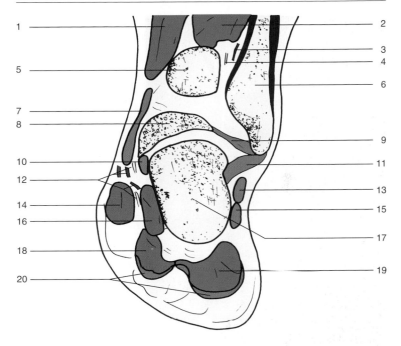

1 Tibialis posterior muscle
2 Flexor hallucis longus muscle
3 Tibialis anterior artery
4 Deep peroneal nerve
5 Tibia
6 Fibula
7 Flexor digitorum longus muscle (tendon)
8 Talus
9 Posterior talofibular ligament
10 Flexor hallucis longus muscle (tendon)
11 Calcaneofibular ligament
12 Medial and lateral plantar arteries, veins, and nerves
13 Peroneus brevis muscle (tendon)
14 Abductor hallucis muscle
15 Peroneus longus muscle (tendon)
16 Quadratus plantae muscle
17 Calcaneus
18 Flexor digitorum brevis muscle
19 Abductor digiti minimi muscle
20 Plantar aponeurosis

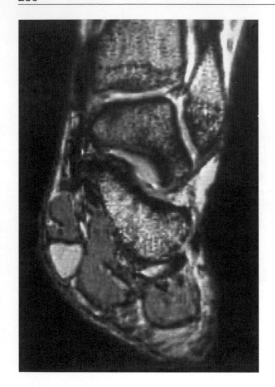

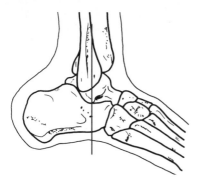

proximal

medial [ ] lateral

distal

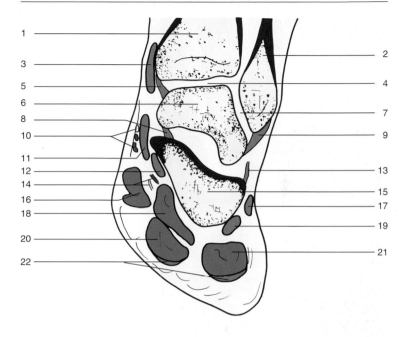

1 Tibia
2 Fibula
3 Tibialis posterior muscle (tendon)
4 Talocrural joint (tibiotalar part)
5 Deltoid ligament (posterior tibiotalar part)
6 Talus
7 Talocrural joint (fibulotalar part)
8 Interosseous talocalcaneal ligament
9 Posterior talofibular ligament
10 Medial plantar artery, vein, and nerve
11 Flexor digitorum longus muscle (tendon)
12 Flexor hallucis longus muscle (tendon)
13 Calcaneofibular ligament
14 Lateral plantar artery, vein, and nerve
15 Calcaneus
16 Abductor hallucis muscle
17 Peroneus brevis muscle (tendon)
18 Quadratus plantae muscle
19 Peroneus longus muscle (tendon)
20 Flexor digitorum brevis muscle
21 Abductor digiti minimi muscle
22 Plantar aponeurosis

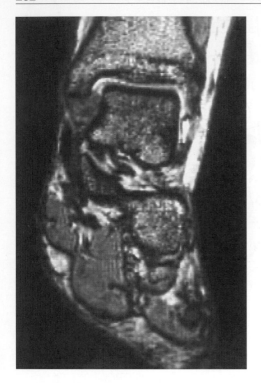

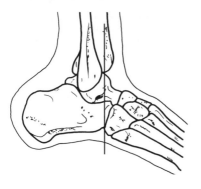

proximal

medial ☐ lateral

distal

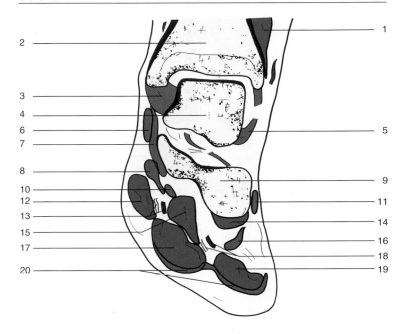

1 Extensor digitorum longus muscle
2 Tibia
3 Deltoid ligament (posterior tibiotalar part)
4 Talus
5 Anterior talofibular ligament
6 Tibialis posterior muscle (tendon)
7 Deltoid ligament (tibiocalcaneal part)
8 Flexor digitorum longus muscle (tendon)
9 Calcaneus
10 Flexor hallucis longus muscle (tendon)

11 Peroneus brevis muscle (tendon)
12 Abductor hallucis muscle
13 Medial plantar artery, vein, and nerve
14 Long plantar ligament
15 Quadratus plantae muscle
16 Peroneus longus muscle (tendon)
17 Flexor digitorum brevis muscle
18 Lateral plantar artery, vein, and nerve
19 Abductor digiti minimi muscle
20 Plantar aponeurosis

234

References

Basset, L. W., R. H. Gold, L. L.
Seeger: MRI Atlas of the
Musculoskeletal System, Deutscher
Ärzte-Verlag, 1989.

Beyer-Enke, S. A., K. Tiedemann,
J. Görich, A. Gamroth: Dünn-
schichtcomputertomographie der
Schädelbasis, Radiologe 27 1987:
438-488

Cahill, D. R., M. J. Orland,
C. C. Reading: Atlas of Human
Cross-Sectional Anatomy.
Wiley-Liss, New York 1990

Chacko, A. K., R. W. Katzberg,
A. MacKay: MRI Atlas of Normal
Anatomy. McGraw-Hill,
New York 1991

El-Khoury, G. Y., R. A. Bergman,
E. J. Montgomery: Sectional
Anatomy by MRI/CT. Churchill
Livingstone, Edinburgh 1990

Feneis, H.: Pocket Atlas of Human
Anatomy. Thieme, Stuttgart 1985

Han-Kim: Sectional Human
Anatomy. Ilchokak, Seoul;
Igaku-Shoin, New York-Tokio 1989

Huk, W. J., G. Gademann,
G. Freidmann: MRI of Central
Nervous System Diseases.
Springer, Berlin 1990

Kahle, W., H. Leonhard, W. Platzer:
Color Atlas and Textbook of
Human Anatomy, Vols. 1–3.
Thieme, Stuttgart 1991

Kang, M. S., D. Resnick: MRI of the
Extremities: An Anatomic Atlas.
W. B. Saunders, Philadelphia 1991

Koritke, J. G., H. Sick: Atlas of
Sectional Human Anatomy.
Urban & Schwarzenberg,
Baltimore–München 1988

Kretschmann, H.-J., W. Weinrich:
Cranial Neuroimaging and Clinical
Neuroanatomy, 2nd ed., Thieme,
Stuttgart 1992

Leblanc, A.: Anatomy and Imaging
of the Cranial Nerves, Springer,
Berlin 1992

Meschan, I.: Synopsis of Radiologic
Anatomy. W. B. Saunders,
Philadelphia 1980

Middleton, W. D., T. L. Lawson (eds.):
Anatomy and MRI of the Joints.
Raven Press, New York 1989

Möller, T. B., E. Reif: MR-Atlas des
muskuloskelettalen Systems,
Blackwell, Berlin 1993

Rauber/Kopsch: Anatomie des
Menschen. Lehrbuch und Atlas.
(Hrsg. H. Leonhardt, B. Tillmann,
G. Töndury, K. Zilles). Band I:
Bewegungsapparat. Thieme,
Stuttgart 1987

Richter, E., T. Feyerabend: Normal
Lymph Node Topography,
Springer, Berlin 1991

Schnitzlein, H. N., F. Reed Murtagh:
Imaging Atlas of the Head and
Spine, Urban & Schwarzenberg,
Baltimore 1990

Stark, D. D., W. G. Bradley:
Magnetic Resonance Imaging,
Mosby, St. Louis 1992

v. Hagens, G., L. J. Romrell,
M. H. Ross, K. Tiedemann: The
Visible Human Body. Lea &
Febinger, Philadelphia 1991

Wegener, O. H.: Ganzkörper-
computertomographie, Blackwell,
Berlin 1992

Witzig, H.: Punkt-Punkt-Komma-
Strich, Falken, Niedernhausen 1991

Index

Acetabulum 199
Achilles tendon 227
Acromioclavicular joint 195
Acromion 187, 195, 197
Aditus ad antrum 33
Amygdaloid body 17, 79, 97
Anulus fibrosus 171, 175
Aorta (bifurcation) 171
Aqueduct 15, 51ff, 73
− (aperture) 103
Arch, vertebral 175
− zygomatic 89ff, 153ff
Arteries
− basilar 19ff, 55ff, 73ff, 99, 141
− carotid (bifurcation) 123, 131
− − common 125ff, 133ff, 145ff, 157
− − external 97, 121, 131, 151, 159
− − internal 19ff, 53ff, 77, 79, 93ff, 117ff,
   131, 145ff, 157ff
− − − (canal) 33
− cerebellar, anterior inferior (AICA) 25
      superior 105
− cerebral, anterior 15ff, 49ff, 91ff
− − middle 17, 77, 79, 95
− − posterior 17, 51, 77, 99ff
− − − (in ambient cistern) 53
− communicating, anterior 17
− − posterior 17, 53
− facial 117, 151
− femoral 199
− genicular, lateral inferior 207ff, 219
− − lateral superior 205ff, 217
− − medial inferior 213ff
− − medial superior 213, 217ff
− humeral circumflex, anterior 187
− − posterior 185ff, 195
− inferior alveolar 143, 151, 153
− infraorbital 89
− insular 15, 81, 93
− maxillary 91, 147, 151
− ophthalmic 89, 91
− pericallosal 45, 99
− plantar, lateral 229ff
− − medial 231ff
− popliteal 209, 221
− posterior choroid 47
− segmental (spinal) 177
− subclavian 159
− subscapular 195

− superficial temporal 117
− suprascapular 183
− tibial, anterior 223, 229
− vertebral 65ff, 77, 79, 97ff, 101, 115ff,
   133ff, 143ff, 159ff
Articular capsule (shoulder) 193
Articular facet 127, 143ff, 175ff
− − C3/4 121
− − C4/C5 123
− − C5/C6 125
− − L2/L3 171
Articular process, inferior 173, 171, 177
− − superior 171, 173, 177
Articular tubercle 83, 17
Articulations/joints
− acromioclavicular 195
− atlantoaxial 161
− atlantooccipital 99, 145, 161
− cricothyroid 137
− talocrural 227, 231
− temporomandibular 61, 151
− − articular disc 31, 83, 179
− tibiofibular 205
− zygapophyseal see articular facet
Atlantooccipital articulation 99, 145
Atlantooccipital membrane, posterior 141
Atlas 35, 143, 163
− and atlantooccipital articulation 161
− (anterior arch) 67, 117, 141
− (lateral mass) 67, 97ff, 101, 115
− (posterior arch) 103
− (transverse process) 81, 147ff
Auditory tube (eustachian) 31, 61ff, 65, 79,
   95, 145
Auditory canal, external 25ff, 61, 149ff, 179
− − internal 23, 33ff, 79, 101
Axis 161
− (arch) 103
− (body) 117ff

Black substance 53, 101
Bones
− cuboid 223ff
− cuneiform, lateral 223ff
− − medial 225ff
− frontal 3ff, 37ff, 43ff, 73ff, 79ff
− hyoid 73ff, 121, 141, 153
− − (body) 131

Bones hyoid (greater horn) 131, 157
- ilium 199ff
- incisive 67
- ischium 201
- metatarsal II 225
- - (base) 227
- metatarsal III 223ff
- metatarsal IV 223
- metatarsal V 223
- navicular 225ff
- occipital 5ff, 19ff, 41ff, 75ff, 79ff, 105ff
- - (external occipital protuberance) 73
- parietal 3ff, 37ff, 51ff, 73ff, 79ff, 93ff
- pubis (inferior ramus) 199
- sacrum 199ff
- - (ala) 203
- sphenoid 19, 23, 51ff, 59, 93, 97, 153
- - (lesser wing) 21
- temporal 13, 17ff, 25, 51ff, 95, 99ff, 105
- - (petrous part) 21ff, 147
- zygomatic 51ff, 83, 87, 151
- - (arch) 65

Calcaneus 223ff
Canal, Bichat's 51
- carotid 31
- facial 31, 33, 101
- mandibular 153, 155
- semicircular 59
- - anterior 57
- - lateral 33ff
- - posterior 33ff, 61
Capsule, external 13, 45ff, 95ff
- extreme 13, 45, 49, 95ff
- internal 45, 49, 77, 79, 93, 97ff
- - (anterior crus) 11ff, 47, 95
- - (posterior crus) 11ff
- - (genu) 13
Carotid bifurcation 123, 131
Cartilage, arytenoid 125, 143
- - (body) 135
- - (vocal process) 135
- cricoid 127, 135, 141ff
- - (Lamina) 137
- retropatellar 207ff
- thyroid 123ff, 135ff, 141, 143, 153
- - (inferior horn) 127, 137
- - (lamina) 133
- - (superior horn) 133ff
Cauda equina 175
- - (in dural sac) 171
Cavity, nasal 57, 61, 87ff, 153ff
- oral 87
- tympanic 25, 35
Cerebellum 73

- caudal lobe 15, 21, 25, 51, 57ff, 103ff, 107
- caudal posterior lobe 63, 81ff, 105
- cranial lobe 15, 51, 53ff
- hemispheres 17ff, 23, 79
- nodule of vermis 57ff
- peduncle 17
- - inferior 23
- - middle 21, 57ff, 103
- pyramis vermis 107
- tonsil 63ff, 75ff
- uvula vermis 61, 73, 105
- vermis 11ff, 17ff, 15, 109
Cerebral peduncle 15, 17, 51ff, 77
Cerebrospinal fluid (postmedullary thecal
    space) 173
Conchae, nasal 65, 75, 87, 89
Choroid plexus 9, 21, 77
Cingulum 7ff, 41, 95
Cistern, ambient 13, 15, 51
- posterior basal 63
- insular 13, 15, 95, 97
- interpeduncular 53, 101
- cerebellomedullary 25, 63, 73ff, 103, 105ff
- cerebellopontine angle 21ff, 57ff
- prepontine 21ff, 61
- quadrigeminal 13, 15, 53
- venae magnae cerebri 51
Claustrum 9ff, 45ff, 95ff
Clavicle 181ff, 189ff
Clivus 19, 25, 59ff, 73ff
Cochlea 31, 59ff, 81ff, 99ff, 147
Colliculus 13
- caudal 53, 73, 103
- cranial 51, 73
Commissure, anterior 49, 73
- - anterior laryngeal 137
- - posterior 73
Confluence of sinuses 57, 141
Conus medullaris 175
Corona radiata 9, 41ff
Corpus callosum 11, 41ff, 103
- (genu) 13, 45, 73, 93
- (splenium) 9, 43ff, 73, 105
- (body) 9, 75, 95ff
Crista galli 19, 51
Cuneus 7ff, 41ff, 51, 107ff

Dorsum sellae 21, 53ff
Duct, nasolacrimal 59ff
- parotid 87, 115, 149ff
- submandibular 87
Dura/dural sac 171, 175

Ear, middle 31
Elastic cone 137
Epidural fat 171, 173ff
Epiglottis 121ff, 131ff, 141ff, 157
– stem 133
Epiphyseal line 205
Esophagus 135ff, 141, 159
Ethmoid labyrinth 25, 51ff, 73ff, 77, 87ff
Eustachian tube 31, 61ff, 65, 95, 145

Falx of cerebrum 3ff, 15ff, 37ff, 87ff, 91ff
– (interhemispheric fissure) 45ff
Fascia, lumbosacral 175
– thoracolumbar 173, 177
Femur 199ff, 209ff, 217
– head 199
– lateral condyle 205ff, 219
– medial condyle 211ff, 219
– neck 199
Fibula 205, 221, 229ff
– (lateral malleolus) 223
Fissure of glottis 135
Fissure, longitudinal 6, 37, 91
– median (central canal) 163
– superior orbital 23, 55, 91, 153
– primary 15
Floccule 25, 59ff, 103
Fluid, cerebrospinal (postmedullary thecal
    space) 173
Fold, aryepiglottic 121, 133
– glossoepiglottic 131
– pharyngoepiglottic 131
– vestibular 125, 133, 141, 157
Foramen magnum 141, 163
Foramen, interventricular (of Monro) 11, 47,
    97
– occipital 141, 163
– intervertebral 173, 177
– lateral aperture of fourth ventricle
    (Luschka's foramen) 61
Fornix 9ff, 97ff
– (anterior column) 47
– (body) 43
– (postcommissural) 49
Fossa, incisive 141
– mandibular 179
– pterygopalatine 145, 153
– retromolar 115
Frontal pole 47

Ganglion, geniculate 35
– trigeminal (gasserian) 57ff, 95
Geniculate body 13
Gland, lacrimal 25, 51, 83

– parotid 63ff, 95, 97ff, 115ff, 131, 151ff,
    159ff
– pituitary 21, 55, 73, 95, 157
– sublingual 75ff, 87, 121, 143
– submandibular 81ff, 119ff, 131, 147ff
– thyroid 127, 135ff, 143ff, 157
Glenoid fossa 181, 191, 195, 197
Glenoid lip, anterior 183
– inferior 195
– posterior 183
– superior 195
Globus pallidus 13, 45ff, 79, 97ff
Gyrus/Gyri
– angular 7, 41ff, 79ff, 107ff
– cingulate 7ff, 43ff, 89ff, 97ff
– frontal 79
– inferior frontal 9ff, 45, 81ff, 89ff
– inferior temporal 15, 19ff, 49ff, 79ff, 97ff
– lateral occipitotemporal 15, 81, 95ff, 105,
    109
– lateral temporal 107
– medial occipitotemporal 79
– middle frontal 5ff, 39ff, 87ff
– middle temporal 11ff, 47ff, 79ff, 93ff
– occipital 7ff, 41ff, 75ff, 79ff, 109
– orbital 17ff, 49, 77, 87ff, 91
– parahippocampal 13ff, 53, 95ff
– postcentral 3ff, 37ff, 75ff, 79ff, 105ff
– precentral 3ff, 37ff, 75ff, 79ff, 97ff
– straight 17ff, 49ff, 87ff
– superior frontal 3ff, 39ff, 75ff, 87ff
– superior temporal 9ff, 43ff, 83, 93ff
– supramarginal 5ff, 41, 81ff, 101ff
– transverse temporal (Heschl's convolutions)
    11, 45, 81, 103

Heschl's convolutions 11, 45, 81, 103
Hippocampus 11ff, 17, 51ff, 79, 99, 105
Humerus 185
– head 181ff, 187, 193ff
– lesser tubercle 183
Hypopharynx 123, 131, 143
Hypothalamus 13ff, 51

Iliotibial tract 199, 217ff
Incus (short crus) 33
– (long crus) 31, 33
Infraglottic space 127, 155
Infrahyoid strap muscles 121ff, 131ff
Infrapatellar fat pad 207ff
Infundibulum (pituitary stalk) 17, 53, 73
Intercondylar eminence 219
Intermediate mass 73
Intertubercular groove 193

Intervertebral disks 141, 159, 171ff,
– (L2/L3) 171
– with intranuclear cleft 175
Ischial tuberosity 203

Joint capsule 213ff, 225
Joint cartilage 205
Joints *see* articulations

Knee
– cruciate ligament 209ff, 219
– joint space 205

Lamina papyracea 87
Laryngeal prominence 135
Larynx 121ff, 133
– (Ventricle) 141, 155
– (Vestibule) 125, 135
Lens 53ff, 79
Ligaments
– alar 161
– calcaneofibular 229ff
– coracoacromial 189, 193
– coracoclavicular 181
– cricothyroid 127
– cruciform (of atlas) 67, 115
– deltoid (tibiocalcaneal part) 233
– – (posterior tibiotalar part) 231ff
– flaval 141, 171ff, 177
– interosseous talocalcaneal 225ff, 231
– interspinal 173
– – (with interspinal bursa) 175
– long plantar 233
– longitudinal, anterior 171ff
– – posterior 141, 161, 171ff
– lumbodorsal 177
– meniscofemoral 209ff
– nuchal 123ff, 141
– patellar 205ff
– plantar calcaneonavicular 227
– supraspinal 173ff
– talofibular, anterior 233
– tibial collateral 217ff
– – posterior 225, 229ff
– tibiofibular, anterior 223
– – posterior 225
– transverse ligament of atlas 73, 117, 141
– transverse ligament of knee 207
– vestibular 155
– vocal 155
Lobe
– insular 9ff, 15, 43ff, 49, 81, 93, 95, 97ff
– temporal 55ff
– – (base) 25, 59

– – (anterior pole) 21, 91
Lobule
– paracentral 3ff, 39, 105
– parietal 39
– – inferior 5
– – superior 3, 107ff
Lung 193
Lymph nodes 151
– anterior jugular 129
– cervical 129
– deep cervical 128, 129
– jugular group, anterior 128, 129
– – inferior 129
– – lateral 128
– nuchal 128, 129
– preauricular 128
– prelaryngeal 129
– pretracheal 129
– retropharyngeal 128, 129
– submandibular 128
– submental 128
– superficial cervical 128, 129
– supraclavicular 129
– thyroid 129

Malleolus, lateral 223
Malleus (handle) 31, 33
– (head) 33
Mammillary body 53, 97
Mandible 65, 79ff, 115, 121, 141ff
– (body) 75ff, 119
– (condyle) 63, 83, 97, 157ff, 179
– (neck) 179
– (ramus) 67, 91ff, 117, 153ff, 157
Mandibular fossa 179
Mastoid air cells 25, 33ff, 179
Mastoid antrum 21, 33ff, 149
Maxilla 63, 75, 87, 143ff
– (alveolar process) 115ff
Meckel's cave 57
Medulla oblongata 25, 61ff, 73, 101, 163
Membrane, thyrohyoid 133
– tympanic 25
Meniscus, lateral (anterior horn) 205ff, 217
– – (intermediate portion) 219
– – (posterior horn) 205ff
– medial (anterior horn) 213ff, 217
– – (intermediate portion) 219
– – (posterior horn) 213ff
Mesencephalic tegmentum 73
Mesencephalon 15, 103
Middle ear 31
Muscles
– abductor digiti minimi 223ff
– – hallucis 229ff

– adductor brevis 199ff
– – longus 199ff
– – magnus 199ff, 203, 215
– arytenoid 141
– – oblique 135
– – transverse 135
– biceps
– – brachii 197
– – – (short head) 183ff
– – – (long head) 181ff, 187ff, 195
– – – (tendon) 181, 183, 187ff
– – femoris 201, 205ff, 219ff
– – – (short head) 203
– – – (long head) 203
– buccinator 143ff
– cervical iliocostalis 127
– constrictor muscle of pharynx 75, 159
– – – inferior 123, 127, 131ff, 137, 145
– – – – with retropharyngeal space 121
– – – middle 141ff
– – – superior 115, 143ff
– coracobrachialis 183ff
– deltoid 181ff
– depressor anguli oris 87, 115, 119ff
– digastric 83, 101, 161
– – (anterior belly) 143ff
– – (intervening tendon) 153
– – (posterior belly) 65ff, 79, 99, 115ff, 151
– erector spinae 171ff
– extensor digitorum brevis 223
– – – longus 205, 217ff, 223, 233
– – – – (tendon) 225
– – hallucis longus 225
– flexor digiti minimi 223
– – digitorum brevis 227ff, 233
– – – longus (tendon) 227ff
– – flexor hallucis longus 225ff
– – – – (tendon) 229ff
– gastrocnemius 211
– – (lateral head) 205ff, 219
– – (medial head) 209ff, 219
– gemellus (tendon) 201
– genioglossus 73ff, 87, 119, 141ff, 153
– geniohyoid 73ff, 121, 131, 141, 153
– gluteus maximus 203
– – medius 199, 201, 203
– – minimus 199
– gracilis 199ff
– – (tendon) 215, 219
– hyoglossus 75, 119, 153ff
– iliac 199
– iliopsoas 199
– infrahyoid strap 121ff, 131ff
– infraspinatus 181, 185, 189ff 197
– – (tendon) 187
– intercostal 183

– interosseous 223, 225
– interspinal 141
– intraocular
– – inferior oblique 81, 87,
– – – inferior rectus 55ff, 79, 87ff
– – lateral rectus 25, 51ff, 79ff, 87ff
– – medial rectus 25, 53ff, 87, 89
– – superior oblique 25, 51, 87ff
– – superior rectus 23ff, 51, 79, 87ff
– latissimus dorsi 185, 189ff, 197
– levator ani 203
– – palpebrae superioris 81, 79, 87ff
– – scapulae 79ff, 119, 123ff, 149ff, 151, 163ff
– – veli palatini 67, 95, 143ff
– longissimus capitis 67, 81ff, 105, 115ff, 121, 149ff, 163ff
– – cervicis 119, 127, 159
– longus capitis 63ff, 75ff, 115ff, 143ff, 149ff, 159
– – colli 79, 119ff, 131ff, 143, 147
– lumbrical 225
– masseter 63ff, 81ff, 89ff, 115ff, 151ff
– mentalis 121
– multifidus 79, 121ff, 145ff, 163ff, 177, 201ff
– mylohyoid 73ff, 119ff, 131, 141ff, 153ff
– oblique, inferior (intraocular) 81, 87,
– – superior 25, 51, 87ff
– oblique, internal (abdominal wall) 199
– obliquus capitis 81, 101
– – – inferior 67, 77, 103ff, 115ff, 143ff, 161ff, 167
– – – superior 103ff, 115, 149, 165
– obturator, external 199ff
– – internal 199ff
– omohyoid 125, 133ff, 155ff
– opponens digiti minimi 225
– orbicularis oculi 87
– – oris 115, 149
– orbital 79
– pectoralis major 185, 189ff
– – minor 185
– – – (tendon) 181
– peroneus brevis 223
– – – (tendon) 229ff
– – longus 217ff, 223
– – – (tendon) 225, 229ff
– piriform 203
– plantar 205ff
– popliteal 207ff, 211
– – (tendon) 205, 217ff
– psoas 171, 199
– pterygoid, lateral 61ff, 79ff, 91ff, 147ff, 179
– – medial 63, 67, 79ff, 91ff, 115ff, 143ff

Muscles quadratus femoris 201
– – lumborum 171, 201ff
– quadriceps femoris (quadriceps tendon)
207, 211, 213
– rectus capitis anterior 63ff
– – – lateralis 81ff, 149
– – – posterior 63, 143
– – – – (major) 65ff, 75ff, 107, 115ff, 145,
149, 167ff
– – – – (minor) 65ff, 75, 107, 167
– – – superior 103
– – femoris (tendon) 209
– – inferior (intraocular) 55ff, 79, 87ff
– – lateral (intraocular) 25, 51ff, 79ff, 87ff
– – medial (intraocular) 25, 53ff, 87, 89
– – superior (intraocular) 23ff, 51, 79, 87ff
– rhomboid 167ff
– sartorius 213, 219ff
– scalene, anterior 121ff, 149ff, 159
– – medial 127, 151, 161
– – posterior 127, 161
– semimembranosus 203, 209ff, 219ff
– semispinalis 165
– – capitis 63ff, 73ff, 107ff, 115ff, 143ff,
167ff
– – cervicis 75ff, 121ff, 127, 143ff, 163, 169
– semitendinosus 203
– – (tendon) 203, 215, 219
– serratus anterior 181ff, 193
– soleus 205ff, 209, 211
– spinalis 123, 127
– splenius capitis 63ff, 75ff, 79ff, 105ff,
115ff, 127, 143ff, 165ff
– – cervicis 119, 127, 147, 163
– sternocleidomastoid 65ff, 99ff, 115ff, 137,
145ff, 155ff
– sternohyoid 79, 123ff, 131ff, 137, 141ff,
155ff
– sternothyroid 123ff, 131ff, 141
– styloid 65, 115ff
– stylopharyngeus 147ff
– subclavius 181ff
– supraspinatus 181, 189ff
– – (tendon) 181, 187, 195
– subscapularis 183ff, 189ff
– temporal 25, 51ff, 79ff, 87ff, 151ff, 179
– – (tendon) 149
– tensor muscle of tympanum 31
– – veli palatini 63, 91, 145
– teres major 185, 189ff, 197
– – minor 183, 187ff, 197
– thyroarytenoid 135
– thyrohyoid 125, 133ff, 143, 155ff
– – (insertion of tendon) 213ff
– tibialis anterior 205, 211
– – – (tendon) 227

– – posterior 219, 227ff
– – – (tendon) 227, 231ff
– trapezius 65ff, 75ff, 79, 83, 115ff, 143ff,
163ff, 173, 181, 189ff
– triceps 187, 189ff, 197
– – – (lateral head) 185
– – – (long head) 185
– vastus intermedius 199, 207
– – lateralis 199ff, 205, 217ff
– – medialis 199, 209ff
– vocalis 135ff
– zygomatic 67
– – major 117

Nasal cavity 57, 61, 87ff, 153ff
– conchae 65, 75, 87, 89
– crest 67
– septum 55, 61ff
Nasopharynx 63, 65ff, 73, 77, 93ff, 115ff,
141, 157
Nerves
– abducens (VI) 25, 59, 89, 91, 93, 95
– facial (VII) 21, 63, 151
– – (first part) 35
– – (second part) 35
– glossopharyngeal (IX) 25, 63, 65ff, 115,
– hypoglossal (XII) 63, 65ff, 117
– inferior alveolar 115, 117, 153
– lingual 115, 153
– mandibular (V/3) 61
– maxillary (V/2) 91, 93
– median 197
– oculomotor (III) 53, 91, 93, 95
– ophthalmic (V/1) 91, 93
– optic (II) 23ff, 51ff, 73ff, 89, 91ff
– peroneal, common 207
– – deep 229
– saphenous 221
– sciatic 201ff
– spinal nerves and roots 119, 143ff, 161,
171ff, 175
– – C2 117
– – L1 177
– – L2 171, 177
– – L3 171
– – S1 177
– tibial 207ff
– trigeminal (V) 23, 57, 101
– – (ganglion) 21
– trochlear (IV) 89, 91, 93, 95
– vagus (X) 25, 63, 65ff, 115, 117, 127
– vestibulocochlear (VIII) 21, 59, 101
Nodule of vermis 57ff
Nucleus, caudate 75ff, 101
– – (head) 9ff, 43ff, 93ff, 99

– – (tail) 9ff
– – (body) 97
– dentate 17ff, 57ff, 75ff
– lentiform 77, 91
– – (putamen, globus pallidus) 101
– red 51, 101

Occipital condyle 65, 97ff, 101, 145, 161
– foramen 141, 163
– pole 11, 47, 57
Occipital protuberance, internal 59
Ocular bulb 23ff, 51ff, 79ff, 87
Odontoid process of axis 67, 73, 97ff, 115ff,
    141, 161
Olfactory tract 89
Operculum, frontal 47, 83
– parietal 83
– temporal 9, 83
Optic chiasm 17, 51, 95
Optic tract 77, 97ff
Oral cavity 87
Orbit 23, 51, 55
– roof 21, 49, 87
Oropharynx 73ff, 77, 119, 141
Ostium of auditory tube (pharynx) 63
Oval window 33

Palate, hard 73ff, 87ff, 117, 141
– soft 91, 141ff, 153ff
Palatine tonsil, 115
Parahippocampus 55
Paralaryngeal space 135ff
Paraspinal fat 171
Patella 207ff
Patellar retinaculum, lateral 205, 215
Peduncle,
– cerebellar 17
– – inferior 23
– – middle 21, 57ff, 103
– cerebral 77
Pes anserinus 215ff
Pharyngeal musculature 157
Pharynx (nasal part) 63, 65, 67, 73, 77, 93ff,
    115, 117, 141, 157
– (oral part) 73ff, 119, 141
– (laryngeal part) 127
Pineal body 11, 49, 73, 103ff
Piriform sinus 121ff, 133ff, 145
Plantar aponeurosis 227ff
Platysma 83, 121ff, 133, 147, 153
Plexus, brachial 127, 151, 181ff, 189ff
– cervical 147ff, 159, 161ff
– choroid 9, 21, 77
– internal vertebral venous 171, 175

Pons 17ff, 55ff, 73ff, 99ff
Precuneus 3ff, 7, 39ff, 75, 107ff
Preepiglottic space 131ff, 155
Process, anterior clinoid 19, 93
– coracoid 181, 189ff
– inferior articular 173, 177
– mamillary 177
– mastoid 31, 63ff, 101ff, 161ff
– palatine 67
– pterygoid 65, 153
– – lateral plate 63, 91
– – medial plate 63, 91
– spinous 119, 171ff
– – L1 175
– – axis 165ff
– styloid 63, 67
– superior articular 171, 173, 177
– transverse 79, 147, 171
– – C1 165
– – C4 161
Promontory 175
Putamen 11ff, 45ff, 79, 93ff, 101
Pyramis vermis 107

Recess, epitympanic 33
– lateral pharyngeal (Rosenmüller's) 65
Reticular formation 55
Retropatellar cartilage 207ff
Retropharyngeal space 141
Rib 145ff, 149ff, 161ff, 181ff, 193, 195
Round window 31

Scapula 183ff, 189, 195ff
– spine 181, 191, 197
Semioval center 5, 39
Septum, nasal 55, 59ff, 87ff, 91
– pellucid 45, 73, 95ff
– precommissural 13
Sinus, cavernous 19ff, 55ff, 73, 93ff, 157
– ethmoid 25, 51ff, 73ff, 77, 87ff
– frontal 17ff, 43ff, 75ff
– maxillary 49ff, 65, 79, 81, 87ff, 143ff, 149
– occipital 17
– piriform 121ff, 133ff, 145
– sigmoid 17ff, 35, 59ff, 83, 103ff, 147, 163
– sphenoid 21, 23ff, 55ff, 75ff, 91ff, 153ff
– straight 9ff, 43ff, 51ff, 73, 107
– superior sagittal 3ff, 37ff, 73, 87ff
– transverse 15, 57, 75ff, 79ff, 107ff, 147
– tympanic 31, 33
Spinal cord 67, 101, 115, 125, 141, 163, 173
– (cervical) 119ff, 127
Spinous process, cervical 141, 165
Stapes 33

Striate body (inferior part) 15
Striate cortex 9ff, 49, 107
Subglottic space 137
Sulcus, calcarine 47, 51, 75, 107ff
– central 3ff, 37ff, 75ff, 79ff, 101ff
– cingulate 7, 73, 89ff
– collateral 13, 53
– lateral 9ff, 43ff, 83, 95ff
– parietooccipital 5ff, 39ff, 49, 73ff
– postcentral 7, 37
– precentral 3ff, 37ff, 81ff
– superior frontal 39
Suprahyoid musculature 131
Suprapatellar bursa 207, 211ff
Suture, coronal 3
– sagittal 3

Talocrural joint 227, 231
Talus 223ff
Tegmentum, mesencephalic 73
Tentorium of cerebellum 13ff, 17ff, 53ff,
　　75ff, 81, 101ff
Thalamus 9ff, 45ff, 75ff, 99ff
– (anterior nuclei) 97
Thecal space 173, 175
Thyrohyoid membrane 133
Thyroid notch, superior 133
Tibia 207ff, 215, 223ff
– condyle, lateral 205
– – medial 211, 213, 221
– plateau
– – lateral 217ff
– – medial 217ff
Tongue 87, 145, 153ff
Tonsil, palatine 115
Tonsil, pharyngeal 141
Trachea 141, 157
Tract, iliotibial 199, 217ff
– olfactory 89
– optic 77, 97ff
Trigeminal (Meckel's) cave 57
Trochanter, greater 199, 203
Trunk, brachiocephalic 159
– sympathetic 121ff
Tube, auditory (eustachian) 31, 61ff, 65, 79,
　　95, 145
Tympanic cavity 25, 35
Tympanic membrane 25

Uncus (of hippocampus) 15, 17, 53, 77
Uvula 73, 141, 157
– and soft palate 117
– vermis 61, 73, 105

Vallecula epiglottica 131, 141
Veins
– axillary 183ff, 191, 195
– basivertebral 171ff
– brachial 189, 197
– cava, inferior 171
– cerebral, internal 49, 73, 103ff
– deep cervical 67, 115, 143ff, 165
– deep occipital 141, 151
– femoral 209
– Galen's 9, 43, 49, 73
– inferior alveolar 153
– infraorbital 89
– jugular 81, 125, 149. 157, 161
– – anterior 131ff
– – internal 65ff, 79, 97ff, 115ff, 127, 131ff,
　　147, 159
– – bulb 33, 63
– ophthalmic 23
– – superior 89
– popliteal 221
– retromandibular 67, 115ff, 159
– saphenous, great 221
– – small 209
Ventricle, (collateral trigone) 9
– fourth 17ff, 55ff, 61, 73
– laryngeal 155
– lateral 7ff, 41, 77ff, 97ff
– – (anterior horn) 9ff, 43ff, 93ff
– – (frontal horn) 43 , 91
– – (posterior horn) 11, 45ff, 105ff, 109
– – (temporal horn) 15ff, 51ff, 79, 97ff, 103
– roof of fourth 103
– third 13ff, 47ff, 73, 97ff, 99ff

Vermis of cerebellum 11ff, 17ff, 15, 109
Vertebral bodies 173
– cervical 159
– C3 131
– C4 121ff, 133ff
– C5 125, 135
– C6 137
– C7 127, 141
– L1 175
– L3 171, 177
– L4 175ff
– S1 175ff
Vertebral body, thoracic 173
Vertebral pedicle 8, 171, 173, 177
Vestibular fold 141
Vestibule (of ear) 33ff
– laryngeal 157
Vocal cord 135, 141, 157